THE
CBD OIL
MIRACLE

**Manage Pain, Improve Your Mood,
Boost Your Brain, Fight Inflammation,
Clear Your Skin, Strengthen Your Heart,
and Sleep Better *with the*
Healing Power of CBD Oil**

LAURA LAGANO, MS, RDN, CDN
INTEGRATIVE CLINICAL NUTRITIONIST
COFOUNDER, HOLISTIC CANNABIS ACADEMY

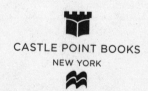

CASTLE POINT BOOKS
NEW YORK

To the women in my family—
my Italian Noni and my mother, Maria Speranza,
whose kitchens informed me about love,
my sister, Carla, who has always been my rock,
and my incredible daughters, Victoria and Isabella,
who have been my best teachers.

www.stmartins.com
www.castlepointbooks.com

The Castle Point Books trademark is owned by Castle Point Publishing, LLC.
Castle Point books are published and distributed by St. Martin's Press.

ISBN 978-1-250-20225-3 (trade paperback)
ISBN 978-1-250-20226-0 (ebook)

Cover design by Young Lim
Interior design by Tara Long
Composition by Christina Gaugler

Images used under license from Shutterstock.com

Our books may be purchased in bulk for promotional, educational,
or business use. Please contact your local bookseller or the Macmillan Corporate
and Premium Sales Department at 1-800-221-7945, extension 5442,
or by email at MacmillanSpecialMarkets@macmillan.com.

First Edition: March 2019

10 9 8 7 6 5 4 3 2

CONTENTS

FOREWORD
CBD CAN CHANGE LIVES

Did you pick up this book because you've heard about CBD, maybe from a friend, a neighbor, or a family member? Or because you're already using and recommending CBD and you want to learn why it works and how else it can help you? Maybe someone suggested that you try CBD. Maybe you have a coworker who started using CBD and you cannot believe how much better he copes at the office. Or you're just curious.

What's up with these three letters, C—B—D?

A lot is the answer. There's a lot happening with CBD and the plant that it comes from, *Cannabis sativa.* Yes, CBD is derived from the cannabis plant—the same plant that provides food with its seeds and whose fiber can be used as a building material. It's the same plant that is the main attraction in marijuana dispensaries—for both medical and adult use—across the country, in Canada, and around the globe. Yes, all these come from *Cannabis sativa.*

When integrated with food, nutrition, aromatherapy, and other holistic modalities, CBD can make a difference—a big difference for some people. Let me be clear: CBD is not a miracle in the sense the term is usually reserved for, as an event that cannot be explained, an unbelievable happening. CBD is not a miracle; it's science, which you'll learn more about in this book. What seems like a miracle, however, is the response that some people have to CBD, the significant impact it can have on day-to-day living—in a good way, as my daughter would say. And that daughter, Isabella, is one of the many people whose life has changed, in part, because of CBD.

Along with a modified ketogenic food plan, targeted supplements, aromatherapy, energy medicine, and a host of other holistic modalities, CBD moved the needle for Isabella. As with some people who use CBD, the needle's movement was not insignificant. That's how I came to CBD. Isabella brought me to the cannabis plant, literally demonstrating the healing properties of this ancient medicine. She showed me how the plant can quell anxiety, help repair the gut, and even improve focus.

Isabella has been my best teacher. A genetic mutation, along with a toxic event (and more), left her with an inability to speak, seizures that were nearly an hour long, delayed development, off-the-wall behaviors, and other issues that prevented her from participating "typically" in life. That's one way to describe autism.

Having become fascinated by the relationship between food and mood, I investigated every nuance of nutrition and brain health. In retrospect, it's crazy that cannabis and CBD never surfaced. How could that be? We know that many individuals who self-medicate with marijuana are dealing with anxiety and insomnia. It turns out that CBD is considered an anxiolytic, meaning an anti-anxiety compound, by the medical establishment—medical professionals in the know, that is.

Throughout my entire journey with Isabella, she taught me how CBD could help her, and I, in turn, taught (or attempted to teach) the special education teachers, doctors, and various therapists in her sphere—of whom there were many. When you have a child with special needs and you want solutions, you never stop looking or educating. It becomes your life mission. Good thing! Without Isabella as my guide, I would not be here to tell you about CBD and its health benefits.

Thank you for joining me—and my daughter—to learn about CBD, health, and wellness. Today, Isabella is training to be a barista and never stops talking.

Laura Lagano
Hoboken, New Jersey
November 29, 2018

CBD is so much more than a supplement to your lifestyle. It may also help manage conditions such as Alzheimer's disease, arthritis, colitis, diabetes, heart disease, osteoporosis, and epilepsy.

THE RISE OF CBD

Balance is a state that everyone seeks in life, yet it can be challenging to achieve. Daily obligations pull us in numerous directions, disrupting our balance. Various areas of life, including work, family, friends, and self-care, among others, frequently become unbalanced. Being in balance feels better, doesn't it?

Could CBD, a compound found in the ancient plant *Cannabis sativa*, help us find that balance? Research scientists, healthcare practitioners, and consumers have reported that cannabidiol, or CBD, may help:

> ➤ Contribute to overall wellness

> ➤ Calm anxiety

> ➤ Relieve chronic pain

> ➤ Reduce overall inflammation

CBD has captured national attention and is rapidly sparking interest around the globe. This cannabis compound has permeated popular culture—in television shows, in articles in magazines and newspapers, online, at your local retailer, basically everywhere. Society is seeking remedies that work in response to the rising costs and scary side effects of healthcare and pharmaceuticals. It seems that CBD is a step in the right direction!

Demystifying CBD, Cannabis, and More

Let's start off by setting the record straight. *Cannabis sativa* refers to the plant itself, both with and without THC. You may already be familiar with the abbreviation THC, for tetrahydrocannabinol, the psychoactive cannabinoid in cannabis. It is historically the most well-known compound found in cannabis.

To simplify, the cannabis community refers to the cannabis plant *with* THC as marijuana and the cannabis plant *without* THC as hemp. More specifically and as defined by the U.S. Farm Bill, marijuana contains more than 0.3 percent THC and hemp contains less than 0.3 percent THC.

CANNABIS *WITH* AND *WITHOUT* THC FOR HEALTH

Did you know that more than half the U.S. states have approved medical marijuana to be sold in dispensaries? Several of those same states have also sanctioned marijuana for adult use. "Adult," rather than "recreational," use is the preferred terminology because many individuals who use cannabis are actually self-medicating—typically for mood disorders, chronic pain, or insomnia. When used properly cannabis is a *healing* plant.

Although CBD can be awesome for health and wellness, cannabis with THC (marijuana) is what started the CBD craze in the first place. Let's be mindful of that. In fact, in some cases, individuals may have better results with medical marijuana than with CBD alone.

STORES AND CLINICS VERSUS DISPENSARIES

CBD from hemp is what you can purchase from healthcare practitioners and at retail stores. You do not need to go to a dispensary for cannabis with CBD, because it contains zero to 0.3 percent THC. The legality of hemp-derived CBD products was previously fraught with debate, but in late 2018, Senate and House agricultural leaders reached an agreement in principle on the 2018 Farm Bill. It's anticipated that hemp will be completely removed from the Controlled Substances Act. (Refer to page 8 for more info.)

CBD from marijuana, or from the cannabis plant containing over 0.3 percent THC (and much higher), can only be purchased in states that have approved medical marijuana or have sanctioned marijuana for adult consumption.

Remember that hemp is the *Cannabis sativa* plant that contains less than 0.3 percent THC. CBD oil, which is what this book is about, can be extracted from either marijuana, the cannabis plant that contains THC, or hemp, the cannabis plant that virtually does not.

Integrating CBD with a Wellness Lifestyle Plan

Integrate CBD with an anti-inflammatory food plan, movement activities, and mindfulness practices and you've created a winning wellness lifestyle plan! With anti-inflammatory and antioxidant properties that rival the most popular lotions and potions, CBD is also primed to become a key player in your beauty routine. Even your pets can benefit from this plant extract.

Yet CBD is so much more than a supplement to your lifestyle. It may also help manage conditions such as Alzheimer's disease, arthritis, colitis, diabetes, heart disease, osteoporosis, and epilepsy. In addition to its antioxidant and anti-inflammatory properties, researchers have found that CBD has amazing anticonvulsant, antidepressant, anti-anxiety, antipsychotic, and neuroprotective qualities.

GETTING STARTED WITH CBD

The CBD market is exploding, which means two things for the consumer. First, you have more products that feature CBD, meaning more ways to incorporate this wellness supplement into your life. You can find oils, gel caps, concentrates, lotions, balms, foods, beverages, sprays, and suppositories that feature CBD for all parts of your body. Second, more choices means more questions and more confusion. Consulting with an integrative healthcare professional who is knowledgeable about CBD before adding the supplement to your routine is recommended.

HOW TO USE THIS BOOK

The following pages will give you a taste of the incredible history of the *Cannabis sativa* plant, a few compounds in cannabis, the healing nature of the plant, and how incorporating CBD into your wellness routine may be beneficial for your health. Learn about CBD products (Practical Products, page 33), general guidelines for using CBD (Dosages and Individualized Medicine, page 38), and how to distinguish CBD products (Be Smart about CBD, page 43). You will also discover the various health conditions for which cannabis may be helpful (Part 2, page 55). And let's not forget the beauty applications of CBD (page 30) and how the plant can help our pets (page 49). There is also a bonus section about the seeds of the cannabis plant—Hemp as Food (page 221).

When you are ready to dive in deeper, meet with a holistic-minded practitioner who can guide you on your journey with CBD and help you navigate the intricacies of your individual biochemistry to achieve balance.

CBD is an antioxidant, anti-inflammatory, anticonvulsant, antidepressant, antipsychotic, antianxiety, and neuroprotectant compound. It's the next big thing in health and wellness.

PART 1

UNDERSTANDING CBD

The Potential of a Plant

ROOTS AND REDISCOVERY

The United States, as a society and a government, seems to have memory loss about cannabis. Officials who have the authority to deschedule cannabis (more on that on page 8) do not seem to appreciate that fewer than 100 years ago the healing power of this plant was well accepted.

Sadly, many people are afraid of the cannabis plant—in both marijuana and hemp form—because of the *cannaphobia,* or fear of marijuana, that persists from the days when Harry Anslinger wielded power. Anslinger was the first commissioner of the U.S. Treasury Department's Federal Bureau of Narcotics. Following Prohibition (of alcohol), he began a propaganda campaign against cannabis and declared that it did more harm than good. He drafted the Marihuana Tax Act of 1937, effectively criminalizing cannabis nationwide. In turn, the act promoted worldwide prohibition against all things cannabis, including hemp, and was the precursor to Nixon's infamous War on Drugs.

Though Anslinger's slanderous claims had no basis, his remarks have influenced the opinions of many Americans—more than 80 years later! Cannabis has a long and dignified history. It was used as

---

Making Connections

To dive deeper into the history of cannaphobia, search for this article online: "Cannaphobia: What's Up with Fear of Marijuana."

---

medicine, for textiles, as building material, and as part of ceremonies for thousands of years. The use of cannabis is not new; society as a whole, which includes scientists and healthcare professionals, is actually rediscovering the capacity of this incredible plant.

Ancient Roots

The cannabis plant first wound its way through the world thousands of years ago, starting in Central Asia before being introduced to Africa, Europe, and then the Americas. At first, people used the plant's seeds as food and its fibers to make clothing, rope, paper, and sails. Ancient cultures knew how to put the rest of the plant to good use, too. China, Egypt, Greece, and India had all incorporated cannabis into their pharmacopeias for conditions such as anxiety, inflammation, and gastro-intestinal issues long before the first century AD. Legend has it that the earliest documented use of *Cannabis sativa* was about 2,600 years ago. Why it was used can only be speculated—possibly medicinal or ritualistic.

A Puritanical Approach

The Puritans of the first American colonies took a more practical approach to cannabis (what a surprise!), using it to make textiles and paper. Hemp was considered so useful and easy to grow that the Virginia, Massachusetts, and Connecticut colonies actually required

Cannabis as Anesthesia

Chinese surgeon Hua Tuo is thought to be the first person to use anesthesia, which included a product containing powdered cannabis called *ma fei san*, though the formula is lost to antiquity. Some historians believe that Hua gave this mixture to his patients in order to perform intense and intricate healing procedures, combining herbal remedies, acupuncture, and surgery to cure even the most difficult conditions, such as brain tumors. He was known as an empathetic surgeon and herbalist who cared deeply for his patients, which is why he experimented with techniques to numb their pain. In fact, the Chinese word for anesthesia literally translates to "cannabis intoxication." Sun Si Miao, an equally well-regarded Traditional Chinese Medicine practitioner, used cannabis leaves topically for relief of pain.

farmers to raise it in the early 1600s. In fact, our founders—including George Washington and Thomas Jefferson—grew hemp on their farms, and the Declaration of Independence and flags made by Betsy Ross were made from hemp! The cannabis plant was intimately part of American life when the colonies were settled.

Americans did not catch up to ancient cultures' use of marijuana as medicine, however, until the late 1800s. While studying in India, Sir William Brooke O'Shaughnessy discovered the healing effects of cannabis. He brought his knowledge to England in the 1830s, and within a few decades the news had spread to the United States, where pharmacies and doctors' offices began to sell cannabis extracts for a multitude of health issues. In fact, cannabis was part of the U.S. Pharmacopeia (USP) from 1850 to 1942 and was once recognized by universities and medical associations as an effective medical treatment for various conditions.

Cannabis was entered into the secondary list of the USP in the third edition of 1850, remained as a primary listing from the fourth entry of 1864 through the 11th edition of 1936, and was removed from the twelfth edition in 1942.

Controlling Cannabis

During the high times of the 1960s, recreational users noticed the health benefits of cannabis with THC. In fact, in 1968 Harvard medical student Andrew Weil (yes, the Andrew Weil who is now a guru of "alternative" medicine) conducted sanctioned research on the effects of cannabis. That same year, over two-thirds of college students in Colorado were in favor of cannabis legalization. Then came the War on Drugs and the Controlled Substances Act of 1970 that classified marijuana as a Schedule I drug—a designation reserved for substances deemed to be addictive and with no medical applications.

According to the Drug Enforcement Agency (DEA), "Schedule I drugs have a high potential for abuse and the potential to create severe psychological and/or physical dependence." Other Schedule I substances include heroin, LSD, and MDMA (known as ecstasy). Interestingly, cocaine, methamphetamine, methadone, oxycodone, and the stimulants Adderall and Ritalin are Schedule II drugs, considered by the DEA to have a lower potential of abuse than cannabis.

That classification prohibited marijuana research; however, scientists continued to take note of anecdotal evidence from cancer and AIDS patients who used the ancient plant medicine for symptom relief.

The First CBD Study

Meanwhile in Israel, Dr. Raphael Mechoulam began conducting research about marijuana and its medicinal potential. He was the first scientist to isolate two of the plant's most important cannabinoids: cannabidiol (CBD) and tetrahydrocannabinol (THC). He also completed the first clinical trial of cannabidiol—a study of CBD's effect on patients with seizure disorders—in which he discovered CBD's anticonvulsant benefits. Years later, Dr. Mechoulam, who is considered the "godfather of cannabis research," identified and named the endocannabinoid anandamide that ultimately led to the breakthrough discovery of the endocannabinoid system. (Learn more about the endocannabinoid system and endocannabinoids on page 20.)

The Promise of Cannabis

Nearly four decades later, we are only beginning to understand the incredible implications of Dr. Mechoulam's work. Thanks to additional cannabis research, scientists have continued to uncover the intricacies of the endocannabinoid system, which—according to the National Institutes of Health—"is one of the most important physiologic systems involved in establishing and maintaining human health." To this day, Dr. Mechoulam speaks on the significance of the system and the ways cannabis can affect humans on a physiological and psychological level. In an interview in *Holistic Primary Care*, he explains that "the

Compassion Wins

California was the first state to advance the case for medical marijuana with the Compassionate Use Act of 1996, which legalized access for people with severe or chronic illnesses. Dozens of states have since followed suit. More and more people are recognizing the amazing potential of THC-containing cannabis in healthcare. Many adults who use marijuana are actually self-medicating. The three most common reasons for cannabis use are anxiety, chronic pain, and insomnia—with or without a medical marijuana recommendation.

Charlotte's Web

Dr. Sanjay Gupta brought the importance of marijuana, cannabis, and CBD to national attention in 2013 with a CNN series called *Weed* that profiled Charlotte Figi, a young girl suffering from a severe form of epilepsy called Dravet syndrome. None of the available conventional treatments made a difference in Charlotte's condition. Her parents watched helplessly as she experienced hundreds of seizures every week, with no end in sight—until they heard about a boy using CBD-rich cannabis oil to reduce his symptoms.

Fortunately for Charlotte, she and her family lived in Colorado, a state that had legalized medical marijuana. They purchased a CBD-rich product from a local medical marijuana dispensary that successfully reduced their little girl's seizures to only a couple per month. That cultivar is now called Charlotte's Web in honor of its brave ambassador.

endocannabinoid system is involved in essentially all human diseases. So obviously, it is of extreme importance." Ultimately, it is all about balance and homeostasis.

Today, scientists and farmers are working to perfect CBD-rich cultivars (known as "strains" in the cannabis-growing world) for numerous health conditions from skin issues to seizures. These are exciting times in the cannabis community: the ancient healing plant is finally regaining its place in the sun, literally!

At a Glance

> Ancient civilizations used the cannabis plant for food, textiles, and medicine.

> Hemp was a major crop when the United States was settled in the 1600s.

> By the late 1800s, American pharmacies were selling cannabis-derived cures, which contained THC.

> The Marihuana Tax Act of 1937 criminalized cannabis following Prohibition.

> The Controlled Substances Act of 1970 halted the use of cannabis entirely—even for medicinal use.

> Dr. Raphael Mechoulam, the "godfather of cannabis research," discovered CBD and THC in Israel and studied their effects on seizure disorders.

> Researchers later identified the human endo-cannabinoid system, which is responsible for balance and homeostasis.

> Scientists are rediscovering the cannabis plant and the medicinal potential of its cannabinoids, including CBD.

BEYOND STIGMA AND CONFUSION

Cannabis is the next big thing in health and wellness, for certain, regardless of whether it contains THC or not. Cannaphobia, however, persists (see Marijuana Is Cannabis, Too, on page 14), and that may leave individuals missing out on the benefits on CBD, THC, and other cannabinoids in cannabis. That is why it is essential to discover and share the findings of integrative healthcare practitioners who are knowledgeable about cannabis and the endocannabinoid system.

A Clear Look at Cannabis

There are a lot of misconceptions about cannabis and its compounds. Here are a few things to keep in mind:

> **CANNABIS WITH LESS THAN 0.3 PERCENT THC,** which is considered hemp, is currently available for purchase.

> **CANNABIS WITH OVER 0.3 PERCENT THC** can be found in states that have medical marijuana dispensaries or permit adult use of marijuana.

> **BOTH THC AND CBD** can be psychoactive—which is why CBD is so great for anxiety and other mood disorders! (Read more about anxiety and depression on pages 73 and 122, respectively.)

> **ONLY THC** can be intoxicating, creating the high.

Keep reading for a deeper exploration of what distinguishes cannabis and its compounds. You can learn more about specific CBD products available in Practical Products, beginning on page 33.

CBD AND THC ARE COUSINS

CBD and THC have a lot in common:

> They both come from the *Cannabis sativa* plant.

> They are each one of more than 100 phytocannabinoids (*phyto-* meaning plant) found in cannabis.

> They both directly and indirectly impact multiple receptor systems in the body.

> They both require decarboxylation from their acids forms, CBDA and THCA, to become CBD and THC, respectively.

> They both have medicinal benefits.

WHAT IS RAW CANNABIS?

It was once believed that it is necessary to *decarboxylate*, or apply heat to, the cannabinoids in cannabis to "activate" them and gain their therapeutic benefits. This has been shown not to be the case; therapeutic value has been demonstrated in the raw cannabinoids in plants that have not been decarboxylated. In fact, some researchers believe that raw cannabinoids may have even more value than their decarboxylated forms for certain health conditions. The most prevalent and significant raw cannabinoids are CBDA (cannabidiolic acid, the raw, nondecarboxylated form of CBD) and THCA (tetrahydrocannabinolic acid, the raw, nondecarboxylated form of THC). These forms of cannabinoids offer unique medicinal properties not always shared by their decarboxylated counterparts. Additionally, the raw form of THC does not have an intoxicating effect.

What Is Decarboxylation?

Technically speaking, decarboxylation is the process by which the carboxyl ring or group (COOH) is removed from cannabinoids. The primary ways this is done are with heat and time. Heating cannabis via vaporization decarboxylates the cannabinoids because the high temperatures make the cannabinoids readily available for absorption. Products labeled as containing CBD have been decarboxylated via heat. Also, over time, as cannabis dries, the raw cannabinoids can slowly and minimally convert to the so-called active forms.

OTHER PHYTOCANNABINOIDS

In addition to CBD and THC, there are over 100 phytocannabinoids in cannabis, each of which communicates differently with the endo-cannabinoid system. Some other well-known phytocannabinoids that are beginning to be investigated include:

> CBC, or cannabichromene

> CBG, or cannabigerol

> THCV, or tetrahydrocannabivarin

> CBN, or cannabinol

MARIJUANA IS CANNABIS, TOO

Because of the stigma attached to the term *marijuana*, many fans of the plant prefer to call it by its scientific name, cannabis. Unfortunately, marijuana is often unjustly associated with intoxication and addiction, and there is a reason for that: propaganda. A 1936 film called *Reefer Madness* depicted cannabis as a highly addictive substance that would lead to hallucinations and criminal behavior. The plant is still often associated with crime and danger and is not fully recognized for its medicinal potential. Be mindful that cannabis with THC—marijuana—has healing benefits, too. Cannabis is not only about CBD.

Discovering the Difference

In the 1970s, marijuana growers started to focus on recreational use, maximizing THC to create the perfect high, so CBD took a back seat for decades. Major milestones in the timeline of discovering CBD were few and far between:

- **1963:** Israeli chemist Raphael Mechoulam began his clinical research on cannabis and isolated the CBD molecule.

- **1980:** Dr. Mechoulam teamed up with South American researchers to publish a study about CBD and epilepsy.

- **1998:** Geoffrey Guy, MD, cofounded GW Pharmaceuticals and joined researchers to develop a CBD pharmaceutical.

- **2003:** Clearly recognizing some potential despite restrictive laws, the U.S. government established a patent for CBD as an anti-inflammatory and neuroprotective!

- **2009:** California's Steep Hill Laboratory tested a cultivar of marijuana provided by Harborside Health Center and found that it had more CBD than THC. Named Soma A-Plus, it was the first CBD-rich cultivar of cannabis in the United States.

Today, many growers are focusing on this key cannabinoid and creating CBD-rich cultivars of cannabis, resulting in the development of a new holistic wellness market.

Better Together

Many cannabis scientists and clinicians believe that the compounds in the plant work better together, not in isolation. This is referred to as the "entourage effect," an idea that was popularized by researcher Ethan Russo. Cannabis contains over 400 compounds, including cannabinoids and terpenes. Different cannabinoids and other plant entities work harmoniously to create therapeutic effects. For example, in some cases, CBD's healing properties are more efficient when THC is also present.

What Is in a Name?

You may think that flowery, silly, and downright strange names like Women's Collective Stinky Purple (one of the first CBD-dominant cannabis plants) are specific to marijuana. Consider that some of your favorite flowers, fruits, and vegetables have unique monikers, too. The person who patents the cultivar gets to name the plant. How about the Pineapple Upside Down Cake hosta, the Hillbilly beefsteak tomato, and Purple People Eater African violets? Now maybe cannabis strains such as Blue Dream, Cannatonic, and Pineapple Express make a bit more sense.

Questions about Cannabis and Feeling High

As a holistic cannabis practitioner who guides clients on integrating cannabis into lifestyle wellness plans, I get asked a lot of questions. Here are the ones most frequently asked, along with answers that give you important information you need in simple terms:

1. **Can you get high using hemp-derived CBD oil?**

   No, you cannot feel the euphoric or intoxicating effects that are possible with CBD's cousin, THC, when using hemp-derived CBD oil. You can, however, experience CBD's anti-anxiety effects, which is why CBD works to modulate mood. (Learn more about these effects in the general discussion that begins on page 19 and in the chapter Anxiety Disorders on pages 73–78.)

2. **If hemp-derived CBD can contain even a small amount of THC, can you fail a drug test?**

   Yes. Although the THC in hemp-derived CBD products is very low (less than 0.3 percent), there is the possibility that THC can be detected in the blood.

3. **If I use a skincare product that contains CBD, will it absorb into my bloodstream?**

   First of all, most skincare products use CBD isolate, so the THC percentage is zero. The amount of CBD that makes it into the bloodstream depends on several factors, such as the type of topical (lotion, cream, balm), other ingredients in the topical, skin thickness, and surface area applied to.

4. **If you use a skincare product with THC, can it be detected in a blood test?**

   Yes, anything that can get through the skin to the bloodstream can be detected in your blood. Again, whether or not it is detected depends on other factors. (See the answer to question 3, above.) Regardless, keep in mind that you cannot count on THC not being detected.

5. **Can you get high from a topical containing THC?**

   Generally, topically applied THC ingredients do not make it into bloodstream in large amounts (compared with oral or inhalation methods), so it is unlikely that you would feel the euphoric effects of THC.

What Is Stopping Us?

Are you wondering, if cannabis—in both medical marijuana and whole plant CBD—has shown health benefits, why is it not more widely accepted and mainstream? There are several reasons:

1. Though cannaphobia is lessening, it is still persistent.

2. Because the federal government designated cannabis as a Schedule I drug—having no medicinal value and high probability for addiction—conducting research on cannabis in the United States is currently illegal, except in rare instances.

3. Most doctors and other healthcare professionals know little or nothing about the endocannabinoid system, phytocannabinoids, and cannabinoids.

With both medical and adult-use marijuana, plus CBD, moving into center stage, however, things are looking good for the *Cannabis sativa* plant! After all, two-thirds of the U.S. states, all of Canada, and other countries around the world have legalized marijuana.

At a Glance

> Tetrahydrocannabinol (THC) and cannabidiol (CBD) are both compounds found in the cannabis plant, called cannabinoids.

> Both THC and CBD confer psychoactive benefits, which is why CBD works to quell mood disorders.

> Only THC can be intoxicating. Though CBD is technically psychoactive, it is not intoxicating.

> Marijuana and hemp are both from the *Cannabis sativa* plant.

> Because the term *marijuana* has negative connotations, many practitioners and researchers prefer the plant's scientific name, cannabis.

> THC and CBD work differently and can be more effective when used together (and with other phytocannabinoids), which is known as the "entourage effect."

> Research into the therapeutic benefits of cannabis would grow exponentially if it were declassified from Schedule I status.

THE SCIENCE BEHIND CBD

Some clinicians think of CBD as a nutrient that our bodies need. The far-reaching impact of CBD and other cannabinoids on the human body is still being discovered by scientists. What we do know is that CBD can promote wellness and treat multiple health conditions.

The Basics

> The cannabis plant features about 400 chemicals, including more than 100 phytocannabinoids such as THC and CBD.

> Cultivars vary by ratios of CBD to THC, which is the most accepted way of indicating the amount of each cannabinoid.

> *Terpenes* are intensely aromatic chemicals that give cannabis its aroma and interact with cannabinoids to impart health benefits. Additionally, terpenes have their own health effects irrespective of interactions. (For more insight on terpenes, see the chart on page 19.)

> Cannabis interacts both directly and indirectly with the endocannabinoid system, which plays a part in just about every bodily process.

> CBD works a little differently in the body than does THC. It indirectly interacts with endocannabinoid receptors by modulating them, as well as using other cell signaling systems such as dopamine, serotonin, glutamate, and GABA—all neurotransmitters.

> CBD also inhibits the breakdown of anandamide, an endocannabinoid produced in the body, making it more available in the brain. (Find more on anandamide on page 20.)

THE ENDOCANNABINOID SYSTEM

Although studies of specific cannabis compounds on the human body are somewhat limited, there was a time when cannabis was at the forefront of U.S. government research. The National Institute on Drug Abuse was trying to prove the negative impacts of cannabis to support the War on Drugs. That is not exactly what happened.

During this research, scientists discovered the endocannabinoid system (ECS), named for the plant that led to the discovery. Working like a lock-and-key system, the ECS is extremely important because it interacts with multiple systems of the body, including the immune, nervous, and digestive systems. By promoting balance and homeostasis, the ECS helps the body adapt to stressors.

CANNABINOID RECEPTORS

The ECS is made up of cannabinoid receptors—referred to as CB1 and CB2—that pick up biochemical cues and affect surrounding cells. CB1 receptors are mainly found in the brain and affect brain development, coordination, movement, learning, sleep, pain, appetite, anxiety, addiction, nausea, and vomiting. CB2 receptors are mainly found in the peripheral nervous system, immune system, gastrointestinal tract, and various organs, including the brain. CB2 activation affects immune responses, such as inflammation, and promotes neuroplasticity, the ability of the brain to form neural connections throughout life.

COMMON TERPENES IN CANNABIS

TERPENE	HEALTH EFFECTS	FOOD SOURCES
Alpha-pinene	Anti-inflammatory, antimicrobial, bronchodilator, neuroprotective	Pine, rosemary, sage
Beta-caryophyllene	Anti-inflammatory, neuroprotective	Black pepper, cardamom, cloves, oregano
Beta-myrcene	Analgesic, anti-inflammatory, sedative	Eucalyptus, hops, lemongrass, mango
Limonene	Anti-anxiety, antidepressant, antimicrobial, antioxidant	Grapefruit, lemons, oranges
Linalool	Analgesic, anti-anxiety, anticonvulsant, antidepressant	Cilantro, coriander, holy basil, lavender

CANNABINOIDS

Cannabinoids are the actual molecules that interact with various receptors in the body—including, but not limited to, CB1 and CB2. *Endocannabinoids* are those produced in the body, anandamide and 2-AG. *Phytocannabinoids* come from plants (hence the prefix *phyto-*), the most well-known being THC and CBD.

HOW DOES CBD WORK?

CBD does not directly bind to the CB1 and CB2 receptors, but it does indirectly influence them. That means the presence of CBD can change the binding of other molecules such as THC and anandamide. That is why a small amount of CBD in cannabis with THC (marijuana) can influence the psychoactivity of THC. Some of the receptor systems that CBD impacts include:

> **SEROTONIN RECEPTORS.** When CBD activates serotonin receptors, it can alleviate anxiety, addiction, appetite loss, insomnia, pain, and nausea.

> **VANILLOID RECEPTORS.** CBD can ease pain and inflammation by activating vanilloid receptors.

> **ORPHAN RECEPTORS.** When the orphan receptor—also known as GPR55—is overactive, it can trigger high blood pressure, osteoporosis, and the spread of cancer cells. CBD can help *deactivate* the GPR55 receptor.

We Make Our Own Cannabinoids

When researchers were looking into how THC affects the brain, they stumbled upon the chemical *anandamide*, or the "bliss molecule," whose name is derived from the Sanskrit word for divine joy, *ananda*. Interacting specifically with CB1 receptors, this endocannabinoid stabilizes mood, relieves pain, and increases well-being. Because THC is structurally similar, it can also trigger the release of feel-good chemicals.

The other major endocannabinoid is 2-arachidonoylglycerol, or 2-AG. One of its functions is to help regulate the immune system. Together, these chemicals are crucial for optimal wellness and disease prevention. They can also assist in disease treatment because of their impact on the major systems throughout the body.

> **NUCLEAR RECEPTORS.** PPARs, or nuclear receptors, regulate energy, insulin, and metabolism and may help stop the progression of Alzheimer's. CBD may help PPARs kick in.

It's All about Homeostasis

Biologist Robert Melamede remarked, "Endocannabinoids are central players in life's multidimensional biochemical balancing act known as homeostasis." Although cannabis or CBD has the potential to improve various health conditions by interacting with numerous systems in the body, it is ultimately all about balance and homeostasis.

In 1998 Vincenzo DiMarzo theorized about the actions of endocannabinoids alone or in combination with other mediators and summed it up by theorizing that some of the messages produced include:

> Relax   > Forget
>
> Eat   > Protect
>
> Sleep

That says it all!

UNDERSTANDING HOMEOSTASIS

Homeostasis means all of your systems are stable, working well, adapting to your needs, and maintaining your body's internal balance. Every system in your body—including nervous, respiratory, digestive, reproductive—requires homeostasis to function optimally. Because all of the systems are connected, a lack of homeostasis in one can create problems in another.

WHY HOMEOSTASIS IS IMPORTANT

Consider this example: When your blood sugar spikes after you eat, your brain signals the release of insulin to regulate it. If this process malfunctions, as it does in diabetes, other organs and bodily processes are affected. One monkey wrench in the works can damage the whole system. In extreme cases, a lack of homeostasis can be deadly.

CLINICAL ENDOCANNABINOID DEFICIENCY AND TONE

In 2001 neurologist Ethan Russo presented a compelling theory of clinical endocannabinoid deficiency (CED), based on the notion that some neurological disorders are associated with neurotransmitter deficiencies. As humans, we have an underlying endocannabinoid *tone*, reflecting levels of the endocannabinoids anandamide and 2-AG. Theoretically, CED can be treated by increasing the production of endocannabinoids, decreasing the breakdown of endocannabinoids, and changing endocannabinoid receptors. In addition to using cannabis or CBD to correct CED, several lifestyle behaviors can affect levels:

> Food and nutrition, or eating habits

> Herbal medicine

> Meditation

> Yoga

> Ayurveda

> Traditional Chinese Medicine

> Movement activities, such as swimming

> Sex with orgasm

> Acupuncture and acupressure

> Qigong

> Massage

Big Pharma Gets Involved

Pharmaceutical companies have taken notice of the healing properties of CBD-rich oil extracts, especially in relation to seizures. The FDA recently approved Epidiolex®, a cannabidiol isolate, for the treatment of Lennox-Gastaut syndrome and Dravet syndrome (two severe forms of epilepsy).

Isolating CBD from the rest of the plant's components ignores the fundamental principle guiding cannabis as medicine—the entourage effect. Scientists believe that the plant's components are far better together than each is alone, and they are confident that changes in national opinion and law will lead to more studies that will reveal the holistic healing properties that cannabis—both with and without THC—has to offer.

At a Glance

> THC and CBD are two of the 100+ cannabinoids contained in the cannabis plant.

> The endocannabinoid system (ECS), which regulates most bodily processes, was discovered as a result of cannabis research.

> The ECS is made up of neural pathways, neurons, receptors, signaling molecules, and enzymes.

> Phytocannabinoids from plants are similar to the body's own endocannabinoids.

> Clinical endocannabinoid deficiency may be a contributing factor in multiple health conditions.

> Your body is constantly seeking balance and homeostasis, and the ECS plays a major role in achieving it.

CBD FOR A
BETTER YOU

Scientists have discovered and are continuing to discover that both cannabis with THC and whole plant CBD are promising treatments for numerous conditions. Plus, cannabis and CBD may also *prevent* those conditions from cropping up in the first place, making it the ultimate wellness supplement. When integrated in a wellness lifestyle plan, CBD may help with chronic inflammation, anxiety, insomnia, pain, skin disorders, and more. At the end of the day, it is all about balance and homeostasis.

How CBD Can Help

Because scientists are still researching the endocannabinoid system, they are continuing to find new applications for cannabis and its cannabinoids, including CBD. The list of conditions that CBD may impact is already a mile long (just check out Part 2: Getting Specific, starting on page 55). Cannabis researchers have labeled CBD a "promiscuous" compound because it is involved in numerous systems and processes in the body to confer therapeutic benefits. Here are a few roles that CBD plays:

- ➤ Antioxidant
- ➤ Anti-inflammatory
- ➤ Anticonvulsant, or anti-seizure
- ➤ Antidepressant
- ➤ Antipsychotic
- ➤ Anti-anxiety
- ➤ Neuroprotectant

BOOST MOOD

Researchers have discovered that when the neurotransmitter serotonin appears in low levels in the brain, individuals experience depressive and anxious symptoms. Mental illnesses such as depression and generalized anxiety disorder are chemical imbalances in the brain. CBD works in a similar way that antidepressants do. It influences specific serotonin receptors so that the chemical messenger cannot be reabsorbed, making it more available in the brain. CBD's potential to enhance serotonin pathways supports its mood-boosting effects. Learn more about how CBD can be part of treatment plans for anxiety and depression on pages 73 and 122, respectively.

RELIEVE PAIN

CBD can affect pain pathways by activating receptors that regulate pain perception and body temperature. CBD can also reduce the inflammation often associated with temporary pain, such as a swollen stubbed toe, and chronic pain, which often results from irritated, sensitized nerves. Mood disorders that involve the serotonin pathway, such as anxiety and depression, are correlated with chronic pain. Because CBD can target both serotonin and pain pathways, it is a multifaceted option for pain sufferers. You can find more information on CBD for chronic pain relief in the chapter beginning on page 113.

CALM INFLAMMATION

Chronic inflammation is a contributing factor in numerous chronic diseases, ranging from Alzheimer's disease to type 2 diabetes. One of CBD's most important capabilities is as a potent anti-inflammatory. In fact, the government has a patent on CBD as an anti-inflammatory! (It is U.S. Patent No. 6,630,507, if you are interested.) You will find more about CBD's anti-inflammatory properties on page 108.

Talk about a Runner's High

If you love cardio, swimming, yoga, meditation, or having an orgasm, you are certainly familiar with the feeling of euphoria. You have to love those endorphins, right? Not so fast. That high feeling is the work of the endocannabinoid system's anandamide molecule—another reason CBD is so great at elevating mood. Dive deeper into a discussion of anandamide on page 20.

HELP HEART HEALTH

Your heart can be affected by conditions such as hypertension, diabetes, obesity, chronic inflammation, and stress. Fortunately, CBD can target each of these contributors. CBD's anti-inflammatory and antioxidant properties help keep the immune system from causing additional damage in response to the heart. Check out the chapter Heart Disease, beginning on page 151, or read the individual chapters linked to heart health factors, such as Diabetes (page 128) and Chronic Inflammation (page 108).

STRENGTHEN BONES

As you age, your bones naturally weaken, which can leave you open to painful fractures and serious breaks. Diminished bone density may be related to clinical endocannabinoid deficiency. (Read more about CED on page 21.) CBD has been shown to strengthen bones and ward off osteoporosis by indirectly activating the endocannabinoid receptors that regulate bone health and even protect against bone loss. You will find information for incorporating CBD into a bone-strengthening wellness plan on page 197.

FEED BRAIN HEALTH

CBD is neuroprotective, which means that it helps reduce damage to the brain—associated with stress, trauma, or illness—and helps generate neurons. Some studies suggest it may keep serious conditions, such as Alzheimer's (see page 71), from developing by changing gene expression to remove the amyloid plaques. New research indicates that it is the removal system, not the plaques themselves, that is the issue in Alzheimer's. There is also evidence that whole plant CBD (in some cases with low-level THC) can also help to treat gut–brain axis disorders, such as autism. You can learn more about the gut–brain relationship and CBD's connection with it on page 74.

BALANCE HORMONES

The up-and-down fluctuation of hormones throughout a woman's reproductive life cycle can sometimes wreak havoc on mood, anxiety, and overall wellness. The endocannabinoid system, endocrine system, and reproductive system are intimately intertwined, underscoring that cannabinoids can provide balance and homeostasis to the reproductive system. The studies and anecdotal clinical evidence about the relationship between women's health and the endocannabinoid system is overwhelming. Learn more information in the Menopause and Prementrual Syndrome chapters starting on pages 173 and 205, respectively.

REGULATE THE IMMUNE SYSTEM

CBD and THC each has its sweet spot, and CBD definitely owns the immune system. Consider the recovery after a fever. Body temperature needs to lower back down to 98.6 degrees Fahrenheit, which happens with the help of the endocannabinoid system.

SOOTHE SKIN CONDITIONS

Many common skin conditions, such as acne and eczema, start with inflammation. Of course, dealing with inflammation is a specialty of CBD. Endocannabinoid receptors are found in abundance in the skin, which is the second-largest organ in the human body (the microbiome being the largest). CBD can inhibit the overactive immune response that leads to red, irritated, and inflamed skin. CBD topicals have shown promising results for a number of skin conditions, which is why CBD skincare products are popping up everywhere. Check out the chapters on acne (page 55), eczema (page 134), and psoriasis (page 210).

BEAT OXIDATIVE STRESS

While the term *antioxidant* probably is not new to you, you may not actually know what antioxidants do. Well, they protect you from

What about Taking Too Much?

CBD has been recognized for its lack of serious side effects, but proceed with caution. When CBD is taken in conjunction with other medications for serious conditions, such as epilepsy or psychotic disorders, it is important to consult your prescribing clinician about interactions. Current research points to tiredness, diarrhea, and changes in appetite as possible side effects of CBD. Furthermore, in some disorders, such as glaucoma, high doses of CBD can make matters worse. More research is needed to understand the possible effects of overconsumption. Overall, CBD has a favorable safety profile, but it is imperative that people with serious health conditions seek guidance from a medical professional before taking CBD.

excessive oxidative stress in your body—from pollution, trauma, chemical irritants, and more—which damages cells and can lead to numerous serious conditions. In fact, CBD is a more powerful anti-oxidant than the go-to vitamins C and E.

Natural Partners for CBD

Because CBD works best with other holistic approaches, it is best to integrate whole plant CBD into your wellness plan. Here are a few other health options to integrate with CBD to supercharge its impact:

> **ANTI-INFLAMMATORY FOOD PLAN.** Think mostly vegetables of all colors and low-sugar fruits, plus detoxifying herbs such as parsley, rosemary, and cilantro, along with selected dairy products and possibly minimal grains. Yes, this can go beyond gluten-free. Consulting with an integrative clinical nutritionist who is a holistic cannabis practitioner is your best bet for guidance.

> **HIGHLY PROCESSED FOOD DETOX.** Cut down on foods that are highly processed, as they contain highly inflammatory ingredients, especially sugar.

> **NUTRITIONAL SUPPLEMENTS.** CBD pairs well with nutritional and herbal supplements, working synergistically to create balance and homeostasis.

> **MEDITATION.** This ancient practice, along with other mind–body modalities like Qigong, has proven time and again to reduce stress, encourage health, and increase overall happiness. Finding just 10 minutes a day to be still and breathe can make all the difference.

> **MOVEMENT.** Simply stepping away from your desk or getting off the couch can do wonders for your body and mind. Incorporating activities as simple as climbing stairs, taking a dip in the ocean, walking on the beach, and hiking in nature can do wonders for your sense of well-being.

> **ESSENTIAL OILS.** Using oils such as lavender, pinene, and limonene can change your mood and outlook. That feeling of calm that you get in a forest is from the pinene oil in the pine trees!

> **COMMUNITY.** At the end of the day, perhaps the most important wellness partner is being part of a vital community and staying clear of toxic relationships.

At a Glance

> ➤ CBD is an antioxidant, anti-inflammatory, anticonvulsant, antidepressant, antipsychotic, anti-anxiety, and neuroprotectant compound.

> ➤ Runner's high is not about endorphins; it is about endocannabinoids!

> ➤ Taking too much CBD can have side effects, and it is essential to understand how certain medications interact with CBD.

> ➤ CBD packs a powerful punch when integrated with other holistic modalities such as an anti-inflammatory food plan, meditation, movement, essential oils, and community interaction and support.

CBD FOR BEAUTY

With its anti-inflammatory and antioxidant properties, CBD can be a spectacular addition to your beauty routine. It seems that new CBD-infused skincare products are being developed around the clock. And for good reason!

What CBD Does for Skin

Although beauty is anything but skin deep, CBD-infused beauty products address most major skin concerns, from puffy eyes to breakouts, by attacking three key skin aggravators.

INFLAMMATION

Puffy eyes, rashes, redness, and acne are all hallmarks of inflammation. Inflammation is the immune system's response to damaged cells and harmful irritants. The endocannabinoid system is involved in the regulation of the immune system, leading researchers to believe that cannabinoids can have astonishing anti-inflammatory effects. When it comes to skin, CBD can reduce inflammation by suppressing the activity of *cytokines*, proteins that typically communicate with immune cells to signal a response.

FREE RADICALS

As you age, your skin can get thinner and lose its elasticity. Free radicals—created by smoke and sun exposure, for example—can accelerate the aging process by damaging your skin. Antioxidants such as CBD may protect your skin from free radicals.

LOSS OF MOISTURE

Staying hydrated is as important to healthy skin as it is to a healthy body. The fat content of the skin, which is crucial to maintaining the barrier that keeps moisture in and irritants out, can break down. Whole plant CBD oil contains fatty acids that are readily absorbed by your skin to enhance hydration.

CBD Products on the Market

It seems that no category is expanding more rapidly than CBD-infused skincare products. The beauty industry has combined CBD with other skin-forward ingredients in various products meant to balance and nourish the skin.

BATH PRODUCTS

Because CBD's main claim to fame is as an anti-anxiety compound, it makes perfect sense to incorporate it into bath products. Manufacturers have combined essential oils, moisturizers, and CBD in a range of bath bombs, soaking salts, and soaps to create the ultimate spa experience—both relaxing and healing.

BODY PRODUCTS

Whether your skin is battling dryness, redness, or irritation, there is a CBD lotion, balm, butter, or salve for you. Most of these are combined with hydrating ingredients such as coconut oil or shea butter infused with essential oils and botanicals.

FACE PRODUCTS

Facial serums, oils, lotions, and sleep masks have all been upgraded and supercharged with the addition of CBD. These new products may reduce redness, puffiness, acne, and signs of aging.

Stress Relief Is Beautiful

One of the biggest benefits of CBD is its ability to reduce anxiety. What contributes to breakouts, rashes, and dark under-eye circles? Stress! Anxiety! Taking an oral CBD supplement every day may help keep stress responses in check.

Eczema Relief

Real eczema relief means taking away both the physical pain and the redness of the condition. Fortunately, CBD succeeds where other eczema treatments often fail. Combine its anti-inflammatory and pain-relief properties with the soothing elements of a moisturizing balm and you have a winning combination. (Check out page 134 for more information on eczema.)

LIP PRODUCTS

Lips need as much care as the rest of your skin—if not more. Hydrating CBD balms may heal chapped lips and keep them supple and primed for whatever. Some companies have even started creating colorful CBD-infused glosses, so stay tuned. Just make certain that the products do not contain any harmful ingredients, such as petrolatum and parabens. (Get a more complete list of ingredients to watch out for on page 35.)

The Future of Beauty

Beauty brands are recognizing the potential of CBD for skin health. As it becomes mainstream and more research is conducted, the industry will continue to find new uses for this cannabinoid. One brand with a CBD-infused mascara has already promised a whole hemp-laden line of cosmetics. This is just the beginning for loving your skin with CBD.

At a Glance

> CBD is anti-inflammatory, which may make it super-effective for combatting many skin disorders.

> As an antioxidant, CBD is more powerful than the beauty-product favorites vitamins C and E.

> CBD's hydrating properties can have anti-aging effects and promote youthful-looking skin.

> CBD works to quell anxiety, which can, in turn, reduce acne, rashes, and dark circles.

> So far, CBD-infused beauty products include moisturizers, masks, serums, salves, lip balms, and bath bombs, with more being developed all the time.

PRACTICAL PRODUCTS

Cannabis—both with and without THC—is always matched to the individual, not to the condition. If you have a specific health condition, it is best to select your whole plant CBD with the guidance of a practitioner who has experience in integrating whole plant CBD with other holistic approaches, including nutrition, essential oils, and mind-body techniques. For overall wellness, you can use the guidelines for evaluating products in Be Smart about CBD (page 43). There are vast differences between CBD brands—buyer beware!

There are numerous ways to take CBD—from tinctures to suppositories and everything in between. Manufacturers seem to be developing new delivery formats at lightning speed.

Oral Products

Oral CBD products include capsules and gel caps, sublingual tinctures and sprays, and edibles. These products vary in their onset, duration, and bioavailability, so it is important to choose a method based on your individual needs.

CAPSULES AND GEL GAPS

One of the most popular CBD formats is capsules or gel caps because pills are a familiar way to take supplements. If you already take nutritional supplements, adding in a CBD capsule or gel cap can be an easy way to integrate CBD into your routine. Keep in mind that because capsules have to pass through the digestive tract, bioavailability is lower.

Oral products that are coated with a substance that prevents break-down in the stomach—called enteric-coated—can be helpful. (See What Is Bioavailability? on page 36.)

SUBLINGUAL TINCTURES AND SPRAYS

CBD extract can be dissolved into an oil, alcohol, or glycerin base, creating a tincture. Typical oils used to make whole plant CBD sublingual tinctures and sprays include medium-chain triglyceride (MCT), coconut, olive, and hemp seed. Taking CBD sublingually, or under your tongue, can be advantageous. Rather than passing through the gastrointestinal system, CBD is absorbed directly into the bloodstream, which increases bioavailability. Place a dose under your tongue and try to hold it there for two minutes.

Edibles

Edibles are foods that have been infused with cannabis. Of course, edibles are oral products, but these innovative CBD-infused foods deserve a section to themselves. Because edibles need to pass through the digestive system, they take a little longer to have an effect and the effects last longer overall. Some edible products infused with CBD include:

- Oils and butters, primarily used in baking and cooking
- Snacks
- Chocolates
- Food bars
- Tea and coffee
- Gummies and caramels
- Lozenges, hard candies, and mints
- Protein powders
- Water and other beverages

CBD Products for Wellness

CBD can be a welcome addition to an overall wellness plan, especially when integrated with other health-promoting lifestyle choices. CBD is *one piece* of a larger holistic health program that can include practices such as mindful eating, movement activities, meditation, and yoga. You will find many condition-specific ideas that partner well with CBD in Part 2, beginning on page 55..

Be mindful when choosing edibles. Although they are easy to use and often delicious, they can sometimes contain unnecessary sugar, preservatives, and artificial flavorings and colorants—all inflammatory ingredients. So apply the same principles for selecting foods to selecting CBD-infused edibles, meaning no or low sugar and no artificial ingredients. And integrate them into your diet carefully: "Start low, go slow" is the motto.

Topicals

Topicals are products that you apply directly on the skin. The first CBD topicals were developed to help alleviate pain and relax muscles and are available in numerous formats. Additionally, CBD topicals are available for skin issues ranging from skin conditions, such as acne and eczema, to beauty and anti-aging products. (See CBD for Beauty on page 30 for more.)

LOTIONS, CREAMS, BALMS, SALVES, OINTMENTS, AND OILS

Added ingredients can make all the difference in a range of topical CBD products. Think about the products that you already purchase for skin health, and make sure that the CBD-infused skin products you choose also feature other skin-healing ingredients. The same is true for pain relief and muscle relaxation products. There are ointments with aloe for inflamed skin, salves with peppermint oil for sore hamstrings, and massage creams with lavender for relaxation. Here are some ingredients to avoid in personal products, according to the Environmental Working Group:

- BHA & BHT
- Formaldehyde
- "Fragrance," which means artificial
- Mineral oil
- Parabens
- Phthalates
- Polyethylene/PEGs
- Propylene glycol
- Retinyl palmitate, retinyl acetate, retinoic acid, and retinol
- Siloxanes
- Sodium lauryl sulfate and sodium laureth sulfate
- Synthetic colors
- Triclosan and triclocarbon
- Toluene

TRANSDERMAL PATCHES

CBD transdermal patches deliver this cannabinoid over four to six hours, making them a great solution for sports injuries, menstrual pain, and migraines. Apply the patch to a venous part of the body for rapid absorption into your bloodstream. One thing to be aware of when it comes to transdermal patches is the additional ingredients present in the patch. Because the epidermis layer of the skin has extremely protective properties and is meant to keep contaminants out, permeation enhancers are needed to carry the CBD molecules across the skin barrier to permit entry into the bloodstream.

Vaporizers

Vaporizing is not smoking! This method allows you to inhale CBD without the deleterious effects of smoking. (See Select Vaporizers Mindfully on page 47 for information.) Because the vapor goes directly into blood circulation through the lungs, the CBD gets to work immediately and with high bioavailability. Though the effects are immediate, they do not last as long as sublingual methods.

Suppositories

Whether you have issues that prevent you from using other CBD products or you just need relief *now*, suppositories for rectal or vaginal

What Is Bioavailability?

Bioavailability refers to how much of a specific compound— CBD in this case—may be available for your body to use. Higher bioavailability means a higher likelihood that the compound gets used by your body. Every compound that you put into your body— including nutrients in foods and supplements, over-the-counter and prescription meds, and cannabis in all formats—has a certain bioavailability. And that *bioavailability is individual*, meaning the bioavailability of the same CBD in the same format is different for different people. Multiple factors contribute to the bioavailability of a CBD product, including the other cannabinoids in the product, stomach acid (or gastric pH), body chemistry, metabolism, gender, age, diet, and environmental factors. This is actually a specialty area of study called pharmacokinetics.

use may be helpful. Suppositories can be appropriate for women's issues, nausea, gastrointestinal issues, and any health concerns for which taking CBD by mouth is not ideal or possible. Because of the nature of the tissue that suppositories interact with, bioavailability is high.

At a Glance

- CBD as medicine is always matched to the person, not the condition.

- Products that are taken under the tongue, such as tinctures and sprays, have high bioavailability.

- Oral products, such as capsules, tinctures, and edibles, must go through the digestive system before making it to the bloodstream.

- Topicals, such as salves, lotions and balms, deliver CBD slowly over the course of four to six hours.

- Patches are great for pain-related conditions.

- Suppositories work for any issues that preclude taking CBD by mouth, and they have high bioavailability.

- Vaporized and nebulized CBD is effective almost immediately, but the effects do not last as long as those of other products.

DOSAGES AND INDIVIDUALIZED MEDICINE

Healthcare in the United States is based on the medical–pharma model of "one drug for one bug." Pharmaceuticals typically work by blunting pathways in the body for effectiveness, which frequently comes with detrimental side effects. Cannabis with THC and whole plant CBD, on the other hand, work by enabling pathways, creating balance and homeostasis. Could the endocannabinoid system and cannabis be the answer to health and wellness? The more practitioners and researchers learn, the more the answer points to yes. The question of how much cannabis each person needs to produce the desired health effect is a bit trickier.

Safety First

CBD is regarded among researchers as a generally safe product because of its lack of dangerous side effects. The most common side effects of CBD among otherwise healthy individuals are fatigue, diarrhea, and changes in appetite. That being said, if you have any health concerns whatsoever, it is important to speak with a healthcare professional competent in cannabinoid medicine before taking CBD. CBD can have harmful drug interactions (see The Grapefruit Rule on page 39) and can even worsen some conditions, such as glaucoma.

The Grapefruit Rule

Although CBD has a great safety profile, it can impact the clearance of other drugs because it is a *P450 inhibitor*—just like grapefruit. That means that it can affect how you metabolize medications such as painkillers, statins, blood thinners, and insulin. Cancer and epilepsy medications may also be affected by the presence of CBD. Always check with your prescribing doctor before adding CBD to your daily regimen if you take any medications. As a general rule, if grapefruit interferes with your meds, CBD probably will, too.

Individualized Medicine

The chapter Practical Products (page 33) reviews the myriad of options available for taking CBD—from familiar capsules and gel caps to suppositories and everything in between. Select CBD products based on *individual* needs, meaning that the dosage, the delivery method, and other factors are personalized for you specifically. There is no one-size-fits-all solution for any given condition. Two similar people with similar conditions can have completely different reactions to CBD delivery methods and dosages. Work under the guidance of a practitioner who is well versed in integrating cannabis into health and wellness.

FIND YOUR SWEET SPOT

CBD products indicate a wide range of dosages on their labels. That is partly because of the biphasic nature (see Less Is More on page 40)) of CBD and partly because different cultivars and different doses work differently for different individuals—even for the same conditions. It is similar to diets—different food plans work for different people with the same conditions. That is partly because of biochemical individuality—a topic for another book!

Finding your specific sweet spot for CBD—the product, delivery format, and dose—can take trial and error. A cannabis clinician can guide you on your journey with cannabis for health and wellness.

GENERAL GUIDELINES

Here are some guidelines to help you get started:

> **GIVE IT TIME.** CBD can have subtle effects, so sometimes changes are not obvious. Other times, particularly for anxiety

relief, CBD's effects can happen very quickly when using sublingual products.

> **SPREAD IT OUT.** Depending on the format and recommended dose, dividing doses throughout the day may be helpful.

> **LAYER PRODUCTS**. Using various CBD formats can be helpful to gain maximum benefits.

> **BE OBSERVANT.** Watch for changes in your mood, sleep, and health condition. Keeping a journal can be helpful.

Less Is More: Start Low and Go Slow

CBD is *biphasic*, meaning it can have two different effects depending on the dose. Typically:

> **A LITTLE CBD** is stimulating.

> **A LOT OF CBD** is sedating.

That sweet spot is key. Think of it like a curve, but the size and slope of the curve depend on the individual. A dose that helps one person focus may make another person's eyelids droop. Taking too much CBD can cause the opposite problem: while a low dose may mellow your mood, a high dose may amplify anxiety. That is why experts suggest to "start low and go slow."

Getting Started, Simplified

Here are a few suggested steps to take when starting out with CBD. Make sure you read through the chapter "Be Smart about CBD" so that you know what to look for—and what to watch out for—in a CBD product. It seems like uncharted territory out there in terms of CBD products.

> **Choose your method.** Pick the delivery method that works for you.

> **Start low.** Sometimes a little bit is all you need, so start with a low dose of CBD. And remember that because CBD is biphasic, taking too much can make it less effective.

> **Talk to your primary care provider.** If you have a primary care physician or other clinician, be sure to keep him or her informed about the supplements you are using, including CBD.

What to Watch For

Though CBD usually does not have serious effects, there are things to be mindful of:

> **DRY MOUTH.** Not everyone experiences dry mouth, but it is the most common side effect of ingesting hemp extracts. Some consider it a small price to pay for relief.

> **DIZZINESS OR FAINTNESS.** Dizziness and faintness may be good indications that CBD is working as a sedative rather than a stimulant.

> **INCREASED ANXIETY.** If you notice stress levels are rising, you may be overdoing it on the dosage or CBD may not be right for you.

> **DRUG INTERACTIONS.** CBD lowers the activity levels of certain enzymes in the P450 detoxification system in the liver. Because that system is responsible for clearing many drugs from the body and activating other drugs, it is important to talk to your pharmacist about potential interactions. See "The Grapefruit Rule" for more info.

Partnering with a Cannabis Clinician

Consulting with a healthcare professional who is well versed in integrating whole plant CBD with holistic modalities is preferable. Professionals who simply replace your medications with CBD are not necessarily working with you to optimize your health. Cannabis is not meant to be a bandage approach. An integrative cannabis clinician can truly guide you on your journey to wellness using CBD and other approaches to influence your overall health.

If your doctor does not know about the endocannabinoid system or does not appreciate holistic medicine, look for a practitioner who does. When it comes to your health, it is essential to explore all different avenues. Western medicine is based on treating symptoms that accompany disease, rather than healing the root cause of an issue. CBD can have powerful medicinal properties, so partnering with a clinician who understands and appreciates the benefits of cannabis is essential.

At a Glance

> CBD is individualized medicine: you need to find your personal sweet spot.

> There is no one-size-fits-all dose. "Start low, go slow."

> Divide your daily dose throughout the day, depending on format and dosage.

> Layer various product formats to fulfill your individual needs.

> CBD is biphasic, which means that it can have the opposite effect at doses at opposite ends of the spectrum.

> Side effects when taking CBD may include dry mouth, dizziness, faintness, and increased anxiety.

> Always check with your prescribing physician or pharmacist before adding CBD if you are taking medication and if you have a complicated condition.

> Partnering with a holistic practitioner to optimize CBD benefits is essential.

BE SMART ABOUT CBD

Deciding to integrate CBD into your lifestyle is an important step on your journey to health and wellness, a smart decision. Now what? How do you decide what type of product you need? What dose and timing are best for you and your specific needs? What are the differences among brands? These are just a few questions to ask as you set out to find your individualized path with CBD.

As with all supplements and personal products, *caveat emptor*—buyer beware. It is up to you as the consumer to know what you are buying. It is that simple *and* that challenging. Reading labels is a must, as is consulting with a healthcare practitioner knowledgeable about cannabis. Doing a bit of research before you buy a product is key, but here is some guidance for getting started.

Whole Plant Hemp Oil

The term hemp oil is a bit confusing (see Know Hemp Oil versus Hemp Oil on page 44). What we are talking about in this book is whole plant CBD oil extract from the hemp flower. Whole plant means that the product contains various cannabinoids, terpenes, and other plant materials, creating the entourage effect. Many products are labeled "whole plant hemp oil" instead of "CBD oil" for that very reason. For products that you consume by mouth, whole plant hemp oil is generally preferred to CBD isolate. For skincare and beauty products, CBD isolate is acceptable.

Know Hemp Oil versus Hemp Oil

Confusing, right? The CBD oil, or extract, that is made from the flower is what this book covers. And then there is hemp seed oil that is used in cooking and on salads. These are two different products made from different parts of the hemp plant. Check out the Hemp as Food section, beginning on page 221, for more about that type of hemp oil. These oils can be easy to differentiate, simply based on bottle size and price. The healing oil with CBD extract and other cannabinoids (known as whole plant) is typically in a smaller bottle with a dropper and costs more per ounce. Hemp oil that is in the food category has a lower price per ounce, similar in price to other cooking and salad oils.

Read the Label

A hemp-derived CBD label, which belongs in the dietary supplement category, can provide a lot of information. Look for:

> Name of the product and company
> Type of CBD—whole plant or isolate
> Milligrams of extract in the total product and per serving
> Source of the plant—organic, sustainable farm or not
> Ingredients listed in descending order of amount
> Supplement facts
> Directions for use and the recommended dosage
> Extraction method used
> GMP, or Good Manufacturing Practices
> Third-party testing verification

Consult with a cannabis practitioner to determine what is important for you specifically.

CHOOSE ORGANIC

Cannabis is a bioaccumulator, meaning it draws toxins from the soil. Any contaminants that are in the soil can be absorbed by the whole cannabis plant. Toxins are absorbed more into the seed than the flower. When CBD is extracted and concentrated, it too will contain pollutants that were present in the soil. So it is important for CBD products to come from plants grown on farms that use organic growing practices, free of pesticides and other harmful chemicals. Unfortunately, some whole plant CBD brands tend to throw the term "organic" around lightly; again, buyer beware. There is currently no USDA certification for organic cannabis.

AVOID ARTIFICIAL OR UNNECESSARY INGREDIENTS

CBD does not require any chemical fillers, additives, preservatives, or flavors. Check the label for harmful ingredients such as:

> Artificial ingredients—colorings, flavorings, sweeteners

> High-fructose corn syrup

> GMOs

> Preservatives

> Thinning agents, such as propylene glycol

AVOID SWEETENERS

Select products that have zero or little sugar. Sugar contributes to inflammation, which is the exact opposite of what you want from a CBD product. Many cannabis edibles contain sugar, so be sure to read labels.

Regenerative Agricultural Practices

Some hemp farmers are using more organic and regenerative farming methods that increase soil health through crop rotation, cover crops, use of compost, and elimination of synthetic chemicals. Conventionally grown hemp, however, uses synthetic fertilizers and may be grown on land previously used for crops that used the herbicide RoundUp, which contains glyphosate. Glyphosate is a health hazard and has been associated with cancer, autism spectrum disorder, and ADHD. Research indicates that glyphosate is harmful to the gut microbiome, impacting the gut-brain axis. That means that certain hemp brands may do more harm than good because of trace levels of glyphosate in the whole plant CBD extract. Together with a cannabis clinician, you can make smart choices. Health begins in the soil, and consumers supporting organic and regenerative farming help create a better planet.

Ask for Lab Tests

Because whole plant CBD products are a totally new category, there is no standardization. CBD's popularity has spiked in recent years and hemp can be legally grown commercially in only a few U.S. states, so a lot of hemp is imported from China and Eastern Europe, where standards may not be enforced, to keep up with demand. Buyer beware. Within the United States, hemp-growing laws vary from state to state where hemp is permitted to be grown, so quality control standards across the board are lacking.

Sometimes it seems like the Wild West, so it is up to the consumer to figure it out. It is vital that the product has been third-party tested and the manufacturer can provide a recent Certification of Analysis, or C of A. Typically, you would need to ask the manufacturer directly for that document. Of course, if you consult with a competent cannabis clinician, he or she can advise you about products and produce a C of A. Lab testing will provide results to ensure that your CBD product is free of contaminants such as bacteria, fungus, heavy metals, mold, pesticides, and solvents.

Weigh Extraction Methods

To obtain whole plant CBD oil from hemp, it needs to be extracted from the plant. Again, buyer beware: not all extraction methods are created equally. Avoid extraction methods that use unsafe solvents, such as butane or hexane, because they could end up in your CBD product. Other, safer extraction methods include:

> **FOOD-GRADE ALCOHOL.** This method utilizes high-grade grain alcohol, or ethanol, to extract cannabinoids, including CBD. Alcohol extraction has been used to process hemp and other botanical plants for centuries. The historic apothecary

Be Aware of Bioavailability

Bioavailability refers to how well a product is absorbed in the body. Not all products and delivery methods are created equal when it comes to this important factor, so consider bioavailability of various CBD product types when deciding what to use. Refer to What Is Bioavailability? on page 36 for more information.

movement in the United States was based on plant extracts in the late 19th century, but fell out of favor with the advent of synthetic pharmaceuticals. Unfortunately, many brands use ethanol from GMO corn and hexane in the extraction process. Hexane is a byproduct of gasoline that is not safe for human consumption. When done properly and with care, alcohol extraction is an excellent method. It works especially well for tinctures taken sublingually and vape cartridges.

➤ **SUPERCRITICAL CO$_2$.** This extraction method involves using carbon dioxide under high pressure and extremely low temperatures. Unwanted waxes and fats, which reduce shelf-life, often remain when using this extraction method. Although it is an easier process than alcohol extraction, supercritical CO$_2$ is not always appropriate.

Keep in mind that different extraction methods are appropriate for different end products. The best scenario for shoppers is to ask the CBD manufacturer about how the cannabis is grown *and* how it is processed.

Select Vaporizers Mindfully

Vape cartridges frequently contain thinning agents such as propylene glycol, which can turn into a carcinogen (meaning: cancer-causing) called formaldehyde when heated. That is the chemical that is used to preserve dead animals—not exactly a good thing to be breathing into your lungs! Also avoid flavoring agents, which can be toxic. Why breathe in toxic chemicals while you are using a product for health and wellness?

It is also important to consider the inner workings, or hardware, of the vaporizer equipment. Currently, all the cartridges on the market are manufactured in China, where, unfortunately, lower-grade materials may be used to cut costs. The most critical part of the cartridge is its heating element, which warms up the CBD oil into vapor. The cheapest cartridges feature a white silica wick, a metal coil, and plastic parts. To avoid the risk of inhaling toxins, it is imperative to avoid such heating elements. There is also a risk that some of the plant-derived ingredients, such as the terpenes, will erode the plastic components within the cartridge—which means that more toxins get into the lungs. When shopping for a CBD vape cartridge, look for a ceramic heating element with a glass and metal body. This ensures that the heating element does not give off any toxins and that there are no degradable plastic components.

Concerning the CBD cartridges, be sure to stay away, far away, from those that contain artificial flavors or propylene glycol, which are both damaging to the lungs. When breathing in CBD vape oil, you should feel comfortable holding your breath for 10 to 15 seconds, as if it were just air. If your lungs are quick to exhale the vapor and you feel harshness and discomfort, it is a sure way to tell that something is wrong with the hardware, the vape oil, or both. Remember to always ask for a full list of ingredients and lab results for pesticides, heavy metals, residual solvents, microbacteria, cannabinoids, and terpenes.

At a Glance

> ➤ Reading labels and doing a bit of research before you buy a CBD product is important.

> ➤ Select whole plant CBD oil extract from the hemp flower, sometimes labeled as whole plant hemp oil or extract, for the healing uses discussed in this book.

> ➤ It is important for CBD products to be free of artificial ingredients, pesticides, and other harmful chemicals.

> ➤ Verify that the product has been third-party tested and the manufacturer can provide a recent Certification of Analysis.

> ➤ Consult with a cannabis practitioner to determine and find what is important for you specifically when selecting a CBD product.

CBD FOR PETS

From anxiety to arthritis, our pets suffer from a lot of the same ailments that afflict humans. Pets are part of the family and they deserve the same love, attention, and care as everyone else in the family. Cannabis provides an option for keeping pets healthy and happy.

How CBD Can Help

All of CBD's antioxidant, anti-inflammatory, anticonvulsant, antitumoral, and neuroprotective qualities seem to work just as well for pets as they do for humans. Giving CBD to pets can be as easy as taking it yourself—using CBD tincture dropped into food or CBD-containing treats available. With a daily supplement, you may be able to prevent and treat various conditions that affect our furry friends.

EASE ANXIETY

Whether your pet has a skittish temperament, reacts to specific triggers such as thunder or fireworks, or suffers from full-blown anxiety, CBD may help calm it. This may be especially good news for pets that suffer from separation anxiety, which can be extremely difficult for the pet and heartbreaking to watch.

TREAT EPILEPSY

Small animals can experience epilepsy and are typically given anti-seizure meds such as phenobarbital and Kappra (generic: levetiracetam). The medications are effective, but come with a cost—often compromising liver function. CBD is a neuroprotectant and has demonstrated effectiveness in mitigating seizures in humans. (Learn more on page 138.) In fact, the FDA recently approved a CBD pharmaceutical for specific seizure disorders for humans. Keep in mind, however, that epilepsy is complicated to treat. CBD does not always work, and what works one day may not work on another day. Sometimes holistic veterinarians integrate CBD with anti-seizure meds. This underscores the importance of working with an animal healthcare practitioner who is competent in cannabis medicine.

RELIEVE PAIN

Watching an animal in pain can be difficult—to say the least. When it comes to pain, CBD works for pets in a similar manner that it does for humans. It can affect pain receptors, decreasing the animal's feelings of pain. As a powerful anti-inflammatory, CBD can reduce chronic pain from inflamed joints in older animals. Because CBD can also balance mood and calm anxiety, which are related to pain perception, this cannabinoid can be doubly helpful in relieving pain.

BATTLE INFLAMMATORY BOWEL DISEASE

If you have ever had a pet with inflammatory bowel disease (IBD), you know that it is no fun for anyone. Not only does your pet feel terrible, but you may need to get intimately familiar with groomers and carpet-cleaning devices. The anti-inflammatory and antioxidant properties of CBD can target the underlying cause of IBD, and reducing inflammation in the gut can relieve the unpleasant symptoms.

CALM CHRONIC INFLAMMATION

Between aging and breed-specific health issues, one of the most common conditions that pets have is joint pain. Because CBD is a

Do Not Share Your CBD

It is important to use pet-specific CBD products to avoid exposing animals to contra-indicated ingredients—stuff they are not supposed to eat. Several foods that humans tolerate and love, such as grapes, raisins, garlic, and, of course, chocolate, are toxic to our four-legged friends. In addition to ingredients, the concentration of CBD tinctures for humans is not always appropriate for animals. With small pets such as cats, the correct concentration is super-critical.

potent anti-inflammatory, it can be used to ease the pain associated with aging joints. CBD can also be helpful for pancreatitis, which frequently afflicts cats and can be fatal. The inflammation triggered by allergies, which pets experience too, can be calmed by CBD to relieve itching and irritation.

MITIGATE DEGENERATIVE DISORDERS

Senior pets can fall victim to the same senility and nerve issues that affect humans. Proven to be neuroprotective, CBD may be able to keep your old friend feeling like a spring chicken for longer.

Choosing a Pet-Specific CBD Product

Many animal lovers treat their pets better than they treat themselves. How about hitting the fast food drive-through for dinner while serving your pet top-of-line pet food—sound familiar? When choosing a product for your pet, make sure you purchase high-quality CBD that is free of artificial ingredients and additives, and is third-party tested and specifically made for pets. See Be Smart about CBD (page 43).

Here are a few guidelines for finding a safe and effective CBD product just for your pet:

> **GO ORGANIC.** Select organic CBD, as well as organic ingredients in edibles. No pesticides or chemicals for your companion!

> **CHOOSE TINCTURES FOR HIGHER DOSES.** Oil tinctures are easy to dose and administer to your pet in food or directly into the mouth. If your animal is dealing with a specific condition, CBD oil may be preferable. When using CBD as medicine for pets, be sure to keep track of dosage and use a high-quality CBD oil. Treats and chews work well for moderate pain or mild anxiety.

> **AVOID UNNECESSARY INGREDIENTS.** Added sugar is not good for either humans or their pets. Stick with wholesome, pet-friendly ingredients without the sweeteners and fillers.

> **INVEST IN QUALITY.** Make certain you buy a high-quality product. You may end up paying more in vet bills than you save on sub-par CBD tincture.

PROCEED WITH CAUTION

Be cautious with cannabis products for pets. Sometimes animals develop urinary tract infections, IBD, and constipation from the use of whole plant CBD products. This may be due to the high plant wax and fat content of the hemp plant and the extraction methods used. Hemp-derived CBD may be used sparingly, not in large doses. CBD derived from the marijuana plant does not appear to have the same side effects, although drowsiness has been reported among some animals after CBD administration.

Dogs have a high number of endocannabinoid receptors in certain parts of the brain, increasing their sensitivity to THC-containing cannabis products. If dogs are exposed to too much THC, they may demonstrate symptoms of static ataxia, which is a neurological dysfunction that produces loss of coordination and other issues. Be sure to consult a holistic veterinarian if you believe that your pet may benefit from cannabis.

At a Glance

> Pets can reap some of the same benefits from CBD that humans can.

> Conditions in which CBD may benefit pets include anxiety, epilepsy, chronic pain, arthritis, chronic inflammation, digestive issues, and degenerative disorders.

> Choose products that are organic, lab tested, and easy to measure, and avoid added sugars and other unnecessary ingredients.

> Use products made specifically for pets and follow the "start low, go slow" dosing motto.

> When treating a pet with a serious condition, be sure to carefully administer CBD oil by tracking dosage under the supervision of a holistic veterinarian.

*You can read through all
of the conditions or flip to the ones
that specifically interest you.
Either way, you'll discover the
incredible potential of cannabis
and its cannabinoids in health
and wellness.*

PART 2

GETTING SPECIFIC

How CBD Can Help *You*

ACNE

> ➤ Acne can trigger painful areas of inflammation and scarring on the face, chest, shoulders, and upper back.

> ➤ Up to 50 million people in the United States suffer from acne.

> ➤ With its anti-inflammatory properties, CBD may reduce the severity of acne and possibly prevent it.

A pimple appears at the worst time, and you rush to the store to find something that will make it go away. Face washes and medicated creams sometimes make overstated claims. You may resort to covering up the blemish as you wait it out. Or worse, you pick and pop until you are left with something even more obvious and painful than before.

Although the occasional breakout is annoying, true acne—with its constant barrage of painful eruptions—is much worse. Treatments range from over-the-counter products to oral medications, all with varying rates of success and side effects. CBD, with its anti-inflammatory and stress-reducing properties, can be an alternative approach for acne.

Inside Acne

You know acne when you see it: areas of red, painful-looking bumps over the face and upper body. But there are two different kinds of acne:

> ➤ **ACNE** refers to whiteheads, blackheads, and pimples. Essentially, each of these bumps is a tiny infection created by oil, dirt, and dead skin cells clogging your pores.

> **CYSTIC ACNE** (also known as inflammatory acne) refers to larger, more inflamed bumps, where cysts have formed deep under the skin. This acne is much harder to treat and can trigger throbbing pain.

As if the bumps themselves were not painful enough, sometimes acne results in physical scarring and may contribute to self-consciousness.

CAUSES

Acne forms when the skin's oil glands (or *sebaceous glands*) produce too much oil (or *sebum*) and block the opening for the gland's hair follicle (the *pore*). Although blocked pores are the culprit, hormones are generally the driving or underlying factor. Hormones stimulate oil production, which leads to clogged pores. Bacteria flourish inside the blocked pores, creating the painful inflammation.

SYMPTOMS

Signs of acne may be obvious, but the actual symptoms vary. An individual may be susceptible to one type of acne or experience both.

> Blackheads are open pores with dark bacteria inside.

> Whiteheads are small white bumps.

> Papules are swollen, red bumps.

> Pustules, or pimples, are pus-filled papules.

> Nodules, or "blind pimples," are solid, painful bumps beneath the skin's surface.

A Real Problem

Although acne may seem like a minor condition, its effects can be painful physically, emotionally, and financially.

> Of the 50 million people in the United States who suffer from acne, about 10 million are left with scars on their faces and bodies.

> Americans spend over $1.4 *billion* a year on acne treatments.

> An incredible 96 percent of sufferers surveyed reported feeling depressed because of their acne. Even worse, 14 percent reported feeling suicidal!

> Cysts are larger, more painful bumps that become inflamed and filled with fluid.

These irritated lumps and bumps can appear anywhere on the face, chest, shoulders, upper back, and buttocks.

Who Is at Risk?

Almost everyone on the planet—95 percent of the population, to be exact—has experienced some form of acne. Sometimes the symptoms are fleeting, and other times they persist for years. A few factors play into who is more likely to be affected, including:

> **AGE.** Because hormones play the biggest role in the formation of acne, adolescents going through puberty are most susceptible, and especially males, whose testosterone is elevated.

> **GENDER.** Thanks to monthly hormonal fluctuations, women are more likely than men to experience acne beyond puberty. Females account for more than 80 percent of cases of adult acne.

> **FAMILY HISTORY.** Newer studies show that there may be a genetic component to acne.

Top Triggers

Acne can pop up at any time for various reasons, including:

> Hormonal changes such as puberty, pregnancy, and menopause

> Stress

> Food sensitivities

> Consuming dairy products that contain hormones

> Eating a processed carbohydrate–laden diet

> Using products that contain endocrine disruptors

> Overwashing the area

> Using too many skin products or using them too frequently

> Touching your face

> Taking anticonvulsants or steroid medications

The CBD Answer

Not only may CBD soothe angry, inflamed skin, but it can also keep acne from forming in the first place. The result is naturally balanced skin. Depending on the severity of the acne, CBD has the potential to clear it completely. At the very least, it prepares the way for other treatments to be more successful.

HOW TO USE IT

The best way to treat acne with CBD is to apply it directly to the affected area in the form of a topical cream or oil. Make sure the topical product does not contain other ingredients that may aggravate the condition, especially those considered toxic endocrine disruptors. Taking a low-dose oral CBD supplement daily may also help, especially if stress is an acne trigger for you. You can slowly work your way up in increments until you find a dose that offers relief.

WHY IT WORKS

CBD is well known for its anti-inflammatory properties. This cannabinoid appears to calm the skin, allowing more effective treatment for the underlying issue—the clogged pores. Sebaceous glands have their own endocannabinoid receptors, making them *receptive* to cannabinoids. Studies show that applying CBD to skin may help regulate oil production.

CBD VERSUS OTHER TREATMENTS

For a condition as common as acne, you would think that the scientists and dermatologists would have the no-fail treatments figured out. But with severity and sensitivity varying from person to person, treatments range from ineffective to dangerous. And how about looking at the

The Truth about Tanning

Some people believe that hitting the tanning bed is a quick and easy way to combat acne, with the added benefit of a sun-kissed glow. However, tanning only masks the redness and may actually worsen breakouts in the end. The UV rays dry your skin, creating only temporary relief. Your body naturally compensates by producing excess oil, which leads to more clogged pores.

underlying causes rather than treating the acne after it happens? Hello, stress reduction!

> Most over-the-counter products contain salicylic acid, which is better suited to a single pimple.

> Benzoyl peroxide treatments and prescription creams can irritate the skin until it burns.

> Oral medications can cause severe side effects, including depression and suicidal thoughts. Plus, these treatments attack the healthy skin as well as the affected area.

Many forward-thinking healthcare practitioners believe that CBD is a preferable option for both preventing and treating acne. One study found that CBD was more efficient in treating acne than one of the most popular prescription treatments. The same study noted that CBD did not affect the normal skin cells surrounding the acne, meaning it only treats what it needs to treat. As a bonus—and perhaps another reason why it may work—CBD can mitigate stress, one of the underlying triggers for acne. (Learn more about CBD for anxiety on page 73.)

Natural Partners for CBD

Although you cannot control whether or not you are predisposed to acne, there are a few things you can do to keep breakouts at bay. Of course, treating your skin with CBD-infused topical products is one great option. But here are a few more:

> **BE GENTLE WITH YOUR SKIN.** Your first instinct may be to fight fire with fire, but often a simple routine including a gentle cleanser, moisturizer, and sun protection is all you need. Harsh products and medications can cause irritation and lead to additional breakouts. And remember to avoid endocrine disruptors!

> **FIND WAYS TO DE-STRESS.** Furrowed brows and worry lines are not the only way your face may show stress—acne flare-ups are another sign. CBD may help you stay more relaxed, but you also need to root out triggers in your day-to-day activities.

> **GET YOUR OMEGA-3 FATTY ACIDS.** Studies have shown that a daily omega-3 fish oil supplement may help reduce acne. And, of course, eating fish that is high in omega-3 fatty acids is

important. One caveat: Be sure to follow the guidelines about selecting supplements that meet clean standards and about avoiding mercury and other toxins in fish.

> **HEAL FROM THE INSIDE OUT.** Your microbiome—that colony of bacteria and other microorganisms in your gut—can affect your skin health. Changing the foods you eat to promote your microbiome, along with selecting an appropriate probiotic, can help reduce acne.

ADDICTION TO SUBSTANCES

> ➤ Addiction is a chronic, progressive disorder that impairs a person's ability to function, work, relate to others, and more.

> ➤ According to 2014 statistics, 21.5 million Americans (aged 12 and older) are addicted to substances, with nearly 80 percent battling alcohol use disorder.

> ➤ Whole plant CBD may be an appropriate treatment for the triggers and negative consequences of addiction, in addition to treating the drug or alcohol addiction issue.

Many people still think of addiction as something that only happens to *other* people—the ones who choose to take drugs or who cannot walk away from the bar before the drinking goes too far. The truth is that addiction has nothing to do with willpower. Although the first sip or cigarette is a choice, the resulting changes in brain chemistry are not.

Street drugs and alcohol are not the only concerns anymore; abuse of prescription medications is growing exponentially. Death rates from opioid addiction are estimated at 115 per day in the United States—a national crisis that makes it more important than ever to find alternative treatments for both pain and addiction. Cannabis may be able to offer help for people in these two critical struggles and hope for their loved ones who are also affected.

Inside Addiction

Addiction, also referred to as substance use disorder, afflicts one in 10 people, but it affects many more than that. Because many individuals cannot stop their addictive behavior even when they see it is causing harm, families and friendships are torn apart by addiction. Now we know that it is a chronic disease affecting the brain. There is no cure, and sufferers often go through cycles of relapse and remission—much like with type 2 diabetes or asthma. But just as with those conditions, addiction can be managed.

CAUSES

Addiction is the result of complex series of chemical reactions in the brain, but the main issue concerns dopamine production. It goes something like this:

- **FIRST,** substances such as psychoactive drugs and alcohol overstimulate the pleasure centers of the brain, creating a surge in dopamine that gives the user a sense of euphoria.

- **THEN** the body produces less and less dopamine to try to balance things out. That leaves the user craving the rush of dopamine and using more or stronger substances to reach it.

- **FINALLY,** searching for the original high becomes a compulsive habit.

A Real Problem

With consequences including self-destructive behavior, damage to relationships, and potential overdose, addiction can easily ruin lives.

- More than a million American teenagers meet the criteria for addiction.
- Roughly 570,000 people die each year in the United States because of substance abuse.
- The United States spends $600 billion annually on addiction in the forms of healthcare, incarceration, crime, and lost productivity.

The fact that addiction can strike anyone at any time makes it all the more essential that we take this health condition seriously and look for better solutions.

Individuals who get into a daily use pattern with many of the drugs of abuse can also become physically dependent upon their drug of choice. And without that drug, of which alcohol may be one, the body goes into withdrawal, causing various symptoms that range from uncomfortable to excruciating. Using again is the only relief, which makes the cycle nearly impossible to break.

The initial changes in the brain are not the only ones. Long-term substance abuse carves new pathways in the areas of the brain that control judgment, decision-making, learning, memory, and behavior control. These changes add to the compulsion, solidifying the addiction.

SYMPTOMS

Symptoms of addiction can be difficult to spot because users get good at ignoring or hiding them. Once the addiction takes hold, however, a noticeable downward spiral of symptoms can include:

> Excessive consumption of a particular substance, despite problems directly related to its use

> Secrecy and solitude

> Anxiety, usually about finding the next fix

> Denial when approached about drug-related problems

> Lack of interest in friends and hobbies

> Hiding stashes of the abused substance

> Taking unnecessary and high risks

> Financial troubles

> Relationship conflicts

The Truth about Prescription Abuse

Thanks to the increase in the marketing and overprescription of medications to treat health conditions, prescription drug abuse is one of the fastest-growing categories of substance abuse. Many people think of prescription medication as safer than other kinds of drugs, yet tens of thousands of people die every year by overdosing on prescription pain relievers alone. Abusing prescription medications can lead to other kinds of substance abuse when the pain relief stops working or the pills run out. Prescription abuse is a serious factor in overall substance abuse.

Who Is at Risk?

Although anyone can fall victim to addiction under the right set of circumstances, a few factors increase the odds:

> ➤ **FAMILY HISTORY.** Alcoholism and drug addiction can be hereditary, so someone with a family history of addiction needs to be much more careful around addictive substances.

> ➤ **MENTAL HEALTH.** People who suffer from anxiety or depression are twice as likely to have a substance-abuse problem.

> ➤ **ENVIRONMENT.** People in unstable living situations, including abusive environments, may be more susceptible to use drugs as an escape, and those surrounded by substance abuse are more likely to fall victim to it. This often includes children whose family members are addicts, students susceptible to peer pressure, and people living in at-risk communities.

> ➤ **TRAUMA.** Trauma such as sexual assault and physical abuse, whether witnessed or experienced firsthand, and resulting in post-traumatic symptoms or chronic pain or both, can increase a person's risk for turning to addictive substances.

The CBD Answer

It takes an immense commitment to change risky behavior and adopt new coping habits to tackle addiction. But it often takes even more than that. A support system is crucial, and anything that can lessen the symptoms of withdrawal and/or curb the cravings is a light at the end of the tunnel. Cannabis—that means with or without THC—is one of only a few alternatives to prescription medications for treating addiction.

HOW TO USE IT

For addiction and withdrawal symptoms, a transdermal patch, which will slowly and evenly distribute the cannabinoids over a period of time (usually eight hours), can be helpful. The use of a vaporizer containing CBD may also be helpful initially to deal with sudden cravings. Always start with the lowest available dose and move up from there until you find one that works for you. And, of course, work with a healthcare practitioner who understands you, addiction, and cannabis.

WHY IT WORKS

CBD is well known as a treatment for nausea, insomnia, anxiety, irritability, headache, and muscle pain—all of which happen to be symptoms of drug and alcohol withdrawal. Taking a CBD supplement may alleviate these symptoms, making it easier to abstain from the substance and focus on rehabilitation.

Additionally, CBD has shown promising results in research studying its effects on cravings themselves. Remember that the role of the endocannabinoid system is to help a person maintain or regain balance, or both. CBD can work with the endocannabinoid system to supplement or enhance this role. Many people with addiction suffer from cue-induced cravings, such as the smoker who reaches for a cigarette after every meal. In one study, researchers administered three daily doses of CBD to heroin addicts and discovered that their cue-induced cravings were diminished not just for those three days, but for seven days after that. CBD has been shown to hinder the neurological reward pathways that trigger addictive behavior. The excitement around CBD's potential to help individuals recover from substance abuse is phenomenal!

CBD VERSUS OTHER TREATMENTS

Treatment of addiction relies heavily on working with therapists, entering a rehabilitation center or program, and/or joining an addiction support group. But some addictions require medication, especially to help with more severe symptoms of withdrawal. Some of these drugs, such as methadone, need to be rigorously monitored by doctors because they themselves have the potential for abuse. CBD can also treat withdrawal symptoms without serious side effects.

CBD for Smokers

A study by University College London found that CBD can also curb nicotine cravings. Researchers gave inhalers to 24 smokers; half contained CBD and half contained a placebo. The smokers were encouraged to use the inhaler anytime they craved a cigarette. In the end, the people given the CBD inhaler smoked 40 percent fewer cigarettes than those given the placebo.

Natural Partners for CBD

Because treatment relies heavily on a person's breaking the cycle, taking CBD for addiction is just one part of the equation. Here are a few other techniques that can be helpful:

> **TALK TO SOMEONE.** Whether you lean on friends and family or you make regular appointments with a therapist, having a support system is crucial for success in treating addiction.

> **WORK THE STEPS.** Many addicts credit twelve-step programs such as Alcoholics Anonymous and Narcotics Anonymous with saving them. Not only do these programs offer a support system of people who have themselves recovered from addiction and hold each other accountable, but they also provide concrete actions a person can take to remain sober.

> **FIND A NEW HOBBY.** Replace a bad habit with a good one, something that you can focus on and pour your energy into. Do more than just begrudgingly pick something. For this step to help, you need to find something that makes you feel rewarded for being involved in it.

> **CREATE BALANCE IN YOUR DAILY LIFE.** Make room for daily meditation, deep breathing, and restorative yoga practices, which can help balance your endocannabinoid system.

> **TAKE A HIKE.** Hiking in nature can be a restorative experience, especially in a pine forest. The pinene—which is a terpene also found in pine trees—provides a calming effect.

> **SELECT A NOURISHING FOOD PLAN.** Many people with substance abuse disorders also abuse addictive food ingredients such as caffeine and sugar. Work with a registered dietitian-nutritionist to create an anti-inflammatory food plan that reduces other addictive substances.

ALZHEIMER'S DISEASE

> ➤ Alzheimer's disease is a progressive neurological condition that affects memory, cognition, and behavior.

> ➤ It is the most common form of dementia, affecting 5.7 million Americans.

> ➤ The anti-inflammatory and neuroprotective aspects of CBD make it an ideal partner for Alzheimer's treatments.

Forgetting where you have laid your keys is a natural part of life, as well as of aging. Alzheimer's disease is more than misplaced keys—it is forgetting the purpose of your key. This devastating neurological condition is both incurable and progressive, and today's treatments only tackle its symptoms. Scientists are turning to the endocannabinoid system for answers. Not only may CBD relieve Alzheimer's symptoms, but researchers are also hopeful that it can unlock the door to treating the underlying illness.

Inside Alzheimer's

In Alzheimer's disease, misfiring in one area of the brain leads to misfiring in another. As the damage spreads, brain cells lose their ability to function and then die off completely, causing symptoms to appear. First there is memory loss, then personality changes, and finally an inability to function day to day. Although people generally live four to eight years after diagnosis, they can live as long as 20 years after. Ninety percent of what we know about Alzheimer's has been discovered in the last 20 years, so scientists are making great strides in learning how to combat the condition. Promising studies involving CBD are the next step in the evolution of Alzheimer's research.

CAUSES

Alzheimer's is a bit of a mystery. Scientists know that the disease is the result of brain cells dying in a fairly predictable pattern, but they do not know what causes the cells to die. Alzheimer's is linked to factors such as age and genetics (see "Who Is at Risk?"), but researchers are still trying to figure out the real trigger.

SYMPTOMS

Alzheimer's works its way through the brain in stages, with a set of symptoms for each area affected:

> **EARLY SIGNS** include trouble remembering new information, because the disease starts in the part of the brain responsible for learning.

> **MIDDLE-STAGE SYMPTOMS** include anger, confusion, disorientation, paranoia, mood swings, and changes in behavior.

> **THE FINAL STAGE** includes difficulty walking, talking, and even swallowing, as well as susceptibility to infections such as pneumonia.

A Real Problem

Alzheimer's affects not just the 5.7 million Americans who suffer from it. The condition, which is nicknamed "the long goodbye," is heartbreaking for friends and family as they watch their loved one disappear before their eyes.

> Alzheimer's is the sixth leading cause of death in the United States.

> From 2000 to 2015, Alzheimer deaths increased by 123 percent.

> Roughly 83 percent of the help given to older adults comes from family, friends, or unpaid caregivers. Alzheimer's accounts for about half of that care.

Who Is at Risk?

Because scientists do not know what causes Alzheimer's, it is difficult for them to pinpoint who is at risk of developing the disease. But they have noticed several indicators, including:

> **AGE.** Aging is the biggest risk factor. The majority of sufferers are over 65 years old, but a small subset suffer from early-onset Alzheimer's disease.

> **FAMILY HISTORY.** Genetics play a huge role in the risk of developing Alzheimer's, so having a parent or sibling with Alzheimer's increases your risk. A person can have the genes associated with Alzheimer's but not develop the disease, meaning that lifestyle can influence the expression of your genetic predisposition. We can alter gene expression, or *epigenetics*, with lifestyle changes such as an anti-inflammatory food plan, movement activities, and targeted supplements, including CBD.

> **ETHNICITY.** Older Latinos and African Americans are more likely than older whites to develop Alzheimer's—1.5 times and twice as likely, respectively.

> **ENVIRONMENTAL TOXINS.** Heavy metals, such as mercury and lead, and chemicals have a devastating effect on brain cells, disrupting connections in their vast interconnected network.

> **CHRONIC VIRAL AND BACTERIAL INFECTIONS.** The inflammation caused by chronic infections takes its toll on overall health, including brain health.

> **DIABETES.** The underlying inflammation leads to brain changes and dementia, often referred to as "type 3 diabetes."

> **HEART PROBLEMS.** Scientists have noticed a connection between heart conditions, including heart disease, high blood pressure, and high cholesterol, and the risk of developing Alzheimer's disease.

Making Connections

Exploring symptoms related to Alzheimer's may be helpful.
You can learn more in the chapters Anxiety Disorders (page 73) and
Insomnia (page 161) .

The CBD Answer

Because CBD has anti-inflammatory, neuroprotective, antioxidant properties, researchers have a feeling that it could help neurodegenerative diseases like Alzheimer's. So far, so good. Newer studies of what role the endocannabinoid system plays in Alzheimer's are calling out the importance of CBD in its treatment and, it is hoped, an eventual cure. What we know now is that CBD seems to alleviate some of the symptoms, especially agitation and aggression.

HOW TO USE IT

To ward off inflammation—into which category neurodegenerative illnesses fall—you can integrate CBD into your wellness routine. It is best to start low and work your way up to your optimal level. Working with a practitioner who understands how the endocannabinoid system interacts with the neurological system is judicious. Because research into CBD's effect on Alzheimer's is ongoing, there is no recommended dosage for someone already afflicted. Taking a daily supplement may provide symptom relief, according to the research so far.

WHY IT WORKS

Among other things, the endocannabinoid system helps regulate learning and memory, neuroinflammation, oxidative stress, neuroprotection, and neurogenesis—all of which are affected by the development of Alzheimer's. Adding a CBD supplement can fortify the endocannabinoid system, and its neuroprotective properties are thought to help prevent the cell death that accompanies Alzheimer's.

CBD VERSUS OTHER TREATMENTS

Because Alzheimer's treatments are limited to prescription medications such as antidepressants and memory enhancers, patient care is often

The Truth about Alzheimer's Meds

No meds treat the disease itself. Instead, patients are often prescribed antidepressants and memory-enhancing drugs to ease the symptoms of Alzheimer's. That's why continued research, like that on the endocannabinoid system's role in the disease, is so important.

more about coping with the disease. Friends, family, and caregivers are told to avoid situations that can trigger confusion or agitation. Patients are told to get enough rest, even though Alzheimer's disrupts sleep patterns. CBD naturally relieves various Alzheimer's symptoms, including insomnia, anxiety, irritability, and restlessness. It is a simple way to address a sea of complicated emotions, side effects, and changes.

Natural Partners for CBD

Making brain health a priority is the most important step in preventing Alzheimer's, and taking a naturally neuroprotective CBD supplement is a great way to help with that. Here are some other things you can do:

> **STAY SOCIAL.** Keeping an active social calendar of friends, family, and activities helps your brain stay young and form new neural connections.

> **EXERCISE MIND *AND* BODY.** Moving your body is just as important to brain health as learning new things and solving puzzles, so get out and take a hike, ride your bike, or go for a walk. Exercise does not need to mean hitting the gym or playing sports, though those work, too!

> **OPTIMIZE NUTRITION.** An anti-inflammatory food plan is vital for brain health. Research has shown that a modified ketogenic diet, featuring restorative fats, high-quality protein, and copious vegetables and fruit can help reduce the risk of Alzheimer's, along with targeted supplements.

ANXIETY DISORDERS

> ➤ About 40 million adult Americans (about 18 percent of the population) suffer from some sort of anxiety disorder.

> ➤ Only about one-third of sufferers seek out treatment, which means nearly two-thirds are suffering unnecessarily.

> ➤ CBD may help the brain function optimally and redirect serotonin to the right places.

The saying goes, "If you are not worried, then you are not paying attention." Everyone gets anxious from time to time, usually for good reason. But when you cannot shake that uneasy feeling, it could be more than natural anxiety—it could be an anxiety *disorder*. Cannabis, which includes CBD, is one of the most promising treatments for anxiety disorders, thanks to its effects on serotonin.

Inside Anxiety Disorders

Worry has been a normal element of survival since the dawn of human existence. It is part of what kept our ancestors from being eaten by lions! But that deep-rooted instinct gets amplified in people who suffer from anxiety disorders. The disorders themselves are varied, involving persistent worry, fear, or stress that interferes with everyday experiences.

CAUSES

The exact cause of anxiety is still a mystery, but researchers think it is a mixture of nature and nurture. Life experience can be just as influential in the development of a disorder as genetics or biology. For example, someone whose father had anxiety can live a great life and still develop it, yet so can someone who has no family history but has suffered a trauma.

Because about 80 percent of our neurotransmitters are produced in the gut, the gut has been referred to as the second brain. This relationship between the gut and the brain means that the food you eat can affect anxiety—and remember the microbiome's role in the gut–brain connection. The endocannabinoid system is intimately involved as well, acting as a mediator in the gut–brain axis.

Many health issues, including low blood sugar, Lyme disease, mold exposure, viruses, and head trauma, cause brain inflammation, which can manifest as anxiety or depression or both.

Top Types of Anxiety Disorders

Anxiety and its recognized disorders come in many forms, but some of the most common include:

> **Generalized anxiety.** This most common type of anxiety is characterized by constant and uncontrollable worry about possible negative outcomes.

> **Separation anxiety.** Separation anxiety covers not just the unwillingness to be parted from a particular person but also the pervasive fear of losing that person.

> **Social anxiety.** More than just introverts, people with social anxiety have a heightened sense of fear in social situations.

> **Panic disorder.** Exactly as it sounds, this disorder strikes with symptoms of panic that seem to come out of nowhere, including sweating, a pounding heart, dizziness, and feeling out of control. When not panicking, sufferers are frequently worried about the potential for panic.

> **Obsessive-compulsive disorder.** With obsessive-compulsive disorder (OCD), anxiety begets anxiety. Intrusively anxious thoughts (obsessions) provoke anxious reactions (compulsions).

SYMPTOMS

Symptoms can vary depending on the exact form the anxiety takes and whether it is mild, moderate, or severe, but they generally include:

> Feeling worried more often than not

> An inability to shake the feeling of worry, despite knowing it is unwarranted

> Needing to feel in control

> Avoiding people or situations

> Being averse to opportunity or risk

Who Is at Risk?

Anxiety is thought to be triggered by a combination of environment, neurological factors, genetics, and life experience, but scientists have found a few common threads:

> **GENDER.** Women are twice as likely as men to suffer from some form of anxiety disorder.

> **FAMILY HISTORY.** Combined with physical and environmental factors, having a close relative who suffers from anxiety can elevate the risk.

> **MEDICAL HISTORY.** Generalized anxiety rarely works alone. Depression, addiction, eating disorders, and irritable bowel syndrome are all typical diagnoses in a person with anxiety. Anxiety can be both a precursor and a result of chronic illnesses such as heart disease.

> **LIFESTYLE CHOICES.** The food you eat, your relationships, how often you are out in nature, your movement or exercise routine, and many other lifestyle factors impact anxiety.

Making Connections

Exploring health conditions related to anxiety may be helpful. You can learn more in these chapters: Addiction to Substances (page 62), Depression (page 122), Heart Disease (page 151), Insomnia (page 161), and Irritable Bowel Syndrome (page 167).

The CBD Answer

Only about a third of anxiety sufferers get help for their disorder, possibly because the available conventional treatments leave something to be desired. Medications frequently do not work and can even make people feel worse. Integrating CBD with a food plan that supports your gut health and microbiome can help you find balance.

HOW TO USE IT

Because the effects of anxiety are constant, using cannabis throughout the day works best. Tinctures are great because the dose can be tweaked as needed. As with any CBD supplement, you can gradually increase your dosage until you discover the amount that works for you. If you are taking any anti-anxiety meds, be sure to speak with your prescribing doctor, as well as with a healthcare professional who understands the endocannabinoid system.

WHY IT WORKS

Researchers think that CBD works in two ways: First, it makes serotonin more available in the synaptic cleft, which has mood-boosting effects. This is the same way that medications called selective-serotonin reuptake inhibitors (SSRIs) treat anxiety. Second, CBD helps the hippocampus (the part of the brain responsible for memory and cognition) generate new neurons, which has been shown to combat anxiety and depression.

CBD VERSUS OTHER TREATMENTS

Anxiety medications can have side effects that range from mild, such as headache and nausea, to more serious, including depression. It

A Real Problem

Anxiety is the most common mental health issue in the United States, affecting about 40 million people. And with its life-altering symptoms, it is an issue we need to take seriously. Anxiety also:

> Costs the United States more than $42 billion a year;

> Puts sufferers at higher risk for addiction and substance abuse; and

> Is thought to be greatly underdiagnosed.

is important to work with a healthcare professional to find the best treatment for you. Keep in mind that the category of meds called benzodiazepine are highly addictive. When some individuals are prescribed "benzos," they develop a tolerance and cannot get off the medication. Rather than alleviating the anxiety, the meds actually contribute to it.

Natural Partners for CBD

The good thing about anxiety is how well it responds to personalized lifestyle medicine. Cannabis works best for anxiety when integrated with other practices:

> **EMBRACE MENTAL HEALTH COUNSELING.** Talk therapy can help you get to the root of your anxieties to reach that "Aha" moment when it all makes sense, and to discover coping mechanisms.

> **OPTIMIZE NUTRITION.** The food you eat affects brain health. In general, select anti-inflammatory foods such as vegetables, herbs, restorative fats, and high-quality proteins. Avoid pro-inflammatory foods such as sugar, gluten, and artificial ingredients. For specific recommendations, seek the advice of a registered dietitian-nutritionist trained in functional medicine.

The Truth about Anxiety

Anxiety is a real problem that can interfere with life in a big way.

> **Social anxiety** can keep people from making friends, going to events, interviewing for jobs, and more because of an all-encompassing sense of fear about what others think.

> **Generalized anxiety** can make individuals overly cautious and afraid to take risks, which means they miss out on opportunities—and that is in addition to feeling constantly overwhelmed.

> **OCD** can prevent individuals from leaving home and interacting because of an inappropriate and excessive focus on tasks such as cleaning and organizing.

The symptoms of anxiety are as real and physical as those of chronic pain or diabetes, and they need to be viewed that way.

> **TAKE PROBIOTICS.** A probiotic supplement can be a great way to feed your microbiome, which influences the gut–brain connection. You can get targeted recommendations from a functional medicine practitioner.

> **PRACTICE YOGA.** Yoga, with its combination of movement and mental respite, has proven itself to be a stellar way to deal with anxiety. That is because you are producing your own endocannabinoids, which make you feel blissful. (For more on how the endocannabinoid system works, refer to page 71.)

> **MEDITATE.** A regular meditation practice, especially in conjunction with yoga and therapy, can help you clear your head and breathe through the anxiety so that you can overcome it. Meditation upregulates your endocannabinoid system so that you produce your own endocannabinoids.

> **MAKE LOVE.** Yes, sex with orgasm feels good, and it can also reduce anxiety! Once again, it is the endocannabinoid system at work, producing internal endocannabinoids.

APPETITE LOSS

> Appetite loss is a symptom of many conditions, from headaches to depression to cancer.

> Over time, appetite loss can lead to malnutrition, a weak immune system, and organ failure.

> CBD can help fight inflammation and stress to boost the appetite.

A scene from a medical drama or an offensive remark can certainly make you lose your appetite. So can some illnesses, as well as treatments for some health conditions. Cancer treated with chemotherapy is perhaps the most well-known health condition that involves appetite loss. Cannabis—both with and without THC—can stimulate appetite.

Inside Appetite Loss

Have you ever tried to force yourself to eat when you were not hungry or did not like what was on the plate? Getting through the meal suddenly becomes a struggle. Food is one of the greatest pleasures in life, but it can become a burden to those who no longer enjoy it.

CAUSES

The list of possible causes of appetite loss is nearly endless and includes everything from a bad mood to life-threatening conditions. It is one of the most common physical responses to stress, trauma, and illness. See Who Is at Risk? and Top Appetite-Affecting Conditions for a few of the most prevalent reasons for losing interest in food.

SYMPTOMS

Obviously, lacking interest in food is the main symptom of appetite loss, but here are a few others you may recognize:

> Anger and irritation (aka "hanger," or hunger + anger)

> Tiredness

> Absentmindedness about mealtimes

> Weight loss

> Cognitive impairment

And that is just the beginning. Go too long without food and your immune system and organs may begin to shut down.

Who Is at Risk?

Although anyone can suffer a loss of appetite, people who have a higher risk include those who have:

> An infection such as the flu

> A cancerous tumor

> Gastrointestinal distress, such as ulcers or inflammation

> Kidney or liver failure

> An eating disorder

> An overactive *or* underactive thyroid

The CBD Answer

In cases like the flu or mono, the appetite usually returns on its own as the body heals. But when getting enough food becomes a chronic problem, CBD can offer a solution.

HOW TO USE IT

Appetite loss is one condition that can be helped by allowing CBD to travel through the digestive tract. Try a daily CBD supplement in the form of a gel cap. As always, start low and work your way up to a higher dose, if needed, until you find your sweet spot. Spreading the dose out over the course of the day can prolong the effects.

WHY IT WORKS

Whether the result of a particular condition, such as tension headaches, or a medical treatment, such as chemotherapy, loss of appetite has a lot to do with neurology, inflammation, and stress. And those happen to be three areas where CBD works wonders. It can help calm the digestive tract and soothe stressed-out neurons.

CBD VERSUS OTHER TREATMENTS

Because appetite loss is sometimes a side effect or symptom, rather than a full-blown condition, adding a CBD supplement is a way to bring balance back to your body while you treat the underlying condition. But when appetite loss becomes serious, as with cancer treatment, doctors tend to turn to progesterone and steroids—both of which can have side effects. For some people, CBD may be able to reduce or even eliminate the need for strong prescription medications.

Top Appetite-Affecting Conditions

When you find yourself missing more meals than not and you have ruled out a response to medication, consider the possibility of one of the following conditions:

> Tension headaches

> Seasonal affective disorder

> Chronic gastritis, which is an inflammatory condition

> Mononucleosis

> Kidney disease

> Depression

> Anxiety

> Pelvic inflammatory disease

> The flu

Some of these conditions can be serious, so make a doctor's appointment if your appetite does not return. Several conditions that affect appetite also respond to CBD, including depression, anxiety, and inflammatory conditions.

The Truth about "Hanger"

You know *when* you are hangry (hungry + angry), but do you know *why*? Here is what happens when lack of food turns into a bad mood:

➤ Without food, your blood glucose levels drop.

➤ Your brain, which desperately needs glucose, starts to malfunction—you cannot concentrate, you misspeak, you get confused.

➤ Your body releases stress hormones, such as adrenaline, to increase your blood glucose.

➤ You get agitated and may respond to others in a not-so-pleasant way.

Natural Partners for CBD

Hunger is a natural biological function, which means that you may be able to help it kick in with a few adjustments.

➤ **EAT FAT AND PROTEIN.** Fat provides satiety, meaning that it makes you feel full. Eating restorative fats with protein, rather than overprocessed carbohydrates such as sweets, bread, and chips, is the best way to avoid blood-sugar fluctuations.

➤ **EAT YOUR LEAFY GREENS.** Greens such as kale, collards, and arugula enhance your body's natural detoxification process.

➤ **SPICE UP YOUR DAY.** Both fennel and caraway can ease digestion and stimulate the appetite. You can simply add the seeds or their oils to either water or food.

➤ **SPACE OUT YOUR FOOD.** If eating three meals a day is not appealing to you, try splitting them up into six smaller meals throughout the day.

ARTHRITIS

> Arthritis affects more than 50 million people with chronic joint pain, swelling, and stiffness.

> The condition is the number-one cause of physical disability in the United States.

> With its pain-relieving and anti-inflammatory properties, CBD may alleviate arthritis symptoms.

Complaining joints may be more than just the aging process. Joint pain, swelling, and stiffness, combined with a limited range of motion, can all indicate a more serious problem: arthritis. At its worst, arthritis pain can make everyday tasks unbearable. Cannabinoids may take the edge off arthritis, possibly eliminating the need for treatments with side effects such as steroids and invasive treatment options such as surgery.

Inside Arthritis

Arthritis is extremely common, and it actually comprises 100 different but related conditions. You may think of it as a natural part of aging, affecting only the oldest among us. In reality, more than 50 million adults of all ages and more than 300,000 children suffer from some form of arthritis. Symptoms range from mildly irritating to disabling.

CAUSES

The two most common types of arthritis are osteoarthritis and rheumatoid arthritis, which are triggered by two different mechanisms:

> **OSTEOARTHRITIS** (aka degenerative arthritis) occurs with a breakdown of articular cartilage from mechanical

means—rubbing of the joint surfaces—or an old injury, perhaps from sports. Cartilage is a smooth tissue that covers the articulating surfaces of bones and facilitates the motion of the bones upon one another. Arthritic changes in the joint occur when cartilage is compromised, resulting in inflammation.

➤ **RHEUMATOID ARTHRITIS** (aka inflammatory arthritis) is an autoimmune disease, occurring when inflammation ravages the joints. It results in a breakdown of cartilage and other joint tissue from the autoimmune attack of the body upon itself. Rheumatoid arthritis can involve organs as a function of the global attack of the body upon itself.

SYMPTOMS

Arthritis symptoms are a tricky bunch—they differ between types of the condition and may come and go. Telltale signs around the joints include:

➤ Pain

➤ Swelling

➤ Stiffness, especially in the morning

➤ Redness

➤ Warmth

➤ Decreased range of motion

➤ Fatigue

Where in your body you feel the pain and stiffness varies. Osteoarthritis tends to affect the lower back, hips, knees, and feet. Rheumatoid arthritis usually affects smaller joints, like those in the hands and feet.

Who Is at Risk?

Because arthritis is considered a normal part of aging, many people—young and old—do not get the help they need. Remember, anyone can suffer from arthritis. The following factors contribute to the risk of developing arthritis:

➤ **GENETICS.** Not only can a family history of arthritis put you at higher risk of suffering from the condition, but certain genes make you more susceptible to environmental risk factors, such as smoking.

➤ **AGE.** Although people of any age can suffer from arthritis, the risk increases with age.

➤ **GENDER.** Women are more likely to suffer from arthritis than men.

- > **OBESITY.** Extra weight puts more pressure on your joints, which can result in arthritis.

- > **INJURY.** If you injure a joint—while playing sports, for example—you are more likely to develop arthritis in that joint.

The CBD Answer

Early and effective treatment is crucial not only to your joint health but to your overall health, because arthritis may affect internal organs via inflammation. CBD can help fight inflammation, giving you an edge to preserve your joints.

HOW TO USE IT

Both oral and topical CBD treatments may work well for arthritis. You can take a tincture or gel cap, as well as applying a CBD-infused cream, lotion, or balm directly to the sore joint. The amount that each person requires for effectiveness is different. Remember, CBD is personalized lifestyle medicine.

WHY IT WORKS

Much of arthritis pain comes from the irritation and inflammation caused by either disappearing cartilage or immune response and inflammation. CBD's anti-inflammatory and pain-relieving properties work diligently to calm the angry joints of those with arthritis.

A Real Problem

If you think that 50 million sounds like a lot of arthritis sufferers, consider this statistic. Predictions indicate that about 78 million people will be diagnosed with arthritis by the year 2040. That is a problem, because:

- > On average, people suffer with the pain of arthritis for two years before they get treatment.
- > People with arthritis are twice as likely to suffer from depression.
- > Having arthritis can put you at risk for other chronic conditions, such as heart disease and diabetes.

Managing arthritis early on is key to keeping this condition from affecting your independent and active lifestyle.

CBD VERSUS OTHER TREATMENTS

Over-the-counter pain relievers are the most common treatment for arthritis, but long-term use comes with its own set of problems, including stomach ulcers and liver damage. Certainly, no one wants to have surgery, but this is unfortunately what many individuals must resort to in the face of severe pain and immobility. CBD decreases inflammation and relieves pain without long-term side effects.

Natural Partners for CBD

The optimal way to deal with arthritis is with personalized lifestyle medicine, which pairs perfectly with CBD.

> ➤ **RUN HOT AND COLD.** A tried and true way to combat joint pain is to apply heat to relax the muscles and increase circulation, and cold to reduce inflammation and numb the pain. Hot showers, hot tubs, heating pads, ice packs, and even bags of frozen vegetables may all do the trick to provide some relief. Be sure not to apply either hot or cold for more than 20 minutes.

> ➤ **MAINTAIN A HEALTHY WEIGHT.** Excess weight is especially detrimental to arthritis sufferers because extra pounds put stress on the joints. Maintaining a healthy weight can do wonders.

> ➤ **KEEP MOVING.** Regular movement can strengthen the joints and the muscles surrounding the joints, helping to stave off arthritis. Keep in mind that excessive exercise can have the opposite effect. Restorative yoga, swimming, walking, and hiking may be enough to keep stiffness and swelling at bay.

Top Three Movement Activities for Arthritis

Move your body with these options:

> ➤ Range-of-motion activities such as bending and straightening your joints
> ➤ Strengthening activities such as resistance bands, free weights, and gentle yoga
> ➤ Low-impact aerobic activities such as walking, easy hiking, bike cruising, and swimming

Go easy and make time to warm up and cool down.

ASTHMA

> ➤ Asthma causes swelling in the airways, which makes breathing difficult.

> ➤ More than 25 million people suffer from asthma.

> ➤ CBD's bronchodilating effect makes it a promising treatment for asthma.

Breathe in. Breathe out. In. Out. People without asthma tend to take the act of breathing for granted. It is so effortless that you do not spend a second thinking about it. But for people with asthma, those easy breaths can be hard to come by. Asthma attacks trigger wheezing, coughing, and a frightening inability to do that very natural thing—breathe. Although inhalers help with attacks, they also have dangerous side effects. CBD is giving asthma sufferers new hope for relief.

A Real Problem

Asthma is often portrayed as a minor affliction in popular culture. With skyrocketing medical costs and sometimes deadly consequences, this condition needs to be taken seriously.

> ➤ Asthma costs the United States more than $80 billion every year in medical costs and productivity loss.

> ➤ More than 3,500 people die from asthma every year.

> ➤ The number of sufferers has been steadily growing since the 1980s. At last count, asthma affects 7.6 percent of adults and 8.4 percent of children in the country.

Inside Asthma

Asthma is one of the country's most common and costly conditions, affecting more than 25 million people across the United States to the tune of several billion dollars. The condition can range from mildly annoying to life-threatening, with a lot riding on prevention of attacks. With CBD's anti-inflammatory properties, researchers believe it can help asthma sufferers catch their breath.

CAUSES

No one knows why some people get asthma and others do not. Some individuals with asthma are more sensitive to triggers. Here is a list of a few categories of asthma:

> **EXERCISE-INDUCED ASTHMA.** These asthma sufferers may need to opt for low impact activities such as walking, bike cruising, or restorative yoga instead of high-impact exercise like cardio-kickboxing.

> **OCCUPATIONAL ASTHMA.** These asthma sufferers should stay away from jobs that involve toxins, noxious fumes, chemicals, and dust. Sometimes toxins do not have noxious odors. Think about perfumes, which can trigger asthma, headaches, and other issues.

> **ALLERGY-INDUCED ASTHMA.** These asthma sufferers want to steer clear of high pollen counts, furry pets, and living spaces with mold issues.

Top Asthma Triggers

Common triggers for individuals with asthma include:

> Airborne allergens

> Respiratory infections

> Cold air

> Stressful situations

> Overexertion

> Irritating fragrances, fumes, and pollutants

> Beta blockers and some over-the-counter pain relievers (aspirin, ibuprofen, and naproxen)

> Foods with sulfites and preservatives

Of course, triggers vary from person to person.

Other categories of asthma include cold-induced, adult-onset, nocturnal, and aspirin-induced.

SYMPTOMS

Typical symptoms of asthma include:

- Shortness of breath
- Coughing
- Tightness or pain in the chest
- Wheezing

The severity and frequency of asthma symptoms depends on the person, individual triggers, and the seriousness of the condition. For example, some sufferers reach for the rescue inhaler daily, while people with exercise-induced asthma may never see symptoms outside of the gym.

Who Is at Risk?

Although almost anyone can develop asthma, having the following can increase the risk:

- Blood relatives with asthma
- Allergies
- Extra weight that interferes with everyday movement activities
- Smoking habit or exposure to secondhand smoke
- A job that involves chemicals, such as hairdressing or manufacturing

The CBD Answer

With its anti-inflammatory and bronchodilation effects, CBD may someday be the gold standard in treatment for asthma. In fact, it is already an immensely promising part of an overall treatment program. In initial studies, CBD has been shown to reduce the frequency and severity of asthma attacks.

HOW TO USE IT

CBD should be used only as a supplement to your other asthma prevention and treatment routines and medications. It is not fast-acting and will not help during an attack. Instead, a daily dose in tincture or capsule form may help to reduce inflammation. Be sure to work with your prescribing practitioner to integrate your asthma meds, if needed, with CBD. As always with CBD, you need to find the dosage that works for you. Of course, individuals with asthma cannot use any smoked or vaped forms of CBD.

WHY IT WORKS

The endocannabinoid system appears to play a major role in lung function. According to studies, CBD may help keep your airways calm by reducing mucus secretions in asthma. This cannabinoid acts as a vasodilator (which may facilitate blood oxygenation) and bronchodilator, while reducing inflammation. CBD's pain-relieving properties may also reduce the discomfort and tightness associated with asthma attacks. The use of CBD and cannabis for asthma requires more study, given the promising effects already demonstrated plus the high incidence of asthma.

CBD VERSUS OTHER TREATMENTS

Without a cure, asthma sufferers rely on actions and medications to manage the condition. Rescue inhalers, which are used to treat infrequent attacks, have a low risk of dangerous side effects. People with more severe asthma, however, frequently turn to long-acting medications with more serious side effects. CBD's ability to soothe the airway may reduce the need for these more powerful medications and offer another treatment option if meds are not providing the desired relief.

The Truth about Asthma Deaths

Although asthma is controllable, 10 Americans die every day from the condition because they did not get the care they needed. The breakdown looks like this:

➤ Asthma kills four times as many adults as children.

➤ Females of all ages are more likely to die from asthma than males.

➤ African Americans are three times as likely to die from asthma as other races.

Researchers hope that CBD will help reduce the number of unnecessary deaths relating to asthma.

Natural Partners for CBD

Most asthma deaths can be prevented with proper treatment and steps to avoid attacks. While taking a CBD supplement may help, you should also:

> **AVOID YOUR TRIGGERS.** Keeping a detailed journal of attacks and the moments surrounding them can help you pinpoint your triggers. Once you do, be sure to avoid them.

> **FOCUS ON YOUR BREATH.** Make a habit of monitoring your breathing so that you notice the early warning signs of an asthma attack and can react immediately. Prevention is key.

> **MAKE WELLNESS A PRIORITY.** Because asthma sufferers are more susceptible to viruses, you want to make sure you are taking care of yourself. Follow an anti-inflammatory food plan, rest often, and steer clear of others who are sneezing and sniffling.

> **OPTIMIZE NUTRITION.** Asthma often travels with eczema, and both are impacted by gut health. Probiotics may be beneficial in lung health related to asthma because of the interconnectedness of the microbiome and the endocannabinoid system.

ATTENTION-DEFICIT HYPERACTIVITY DISORDER

> Attention-deficit hyperactivity disorder is a chronic condition that affects focus and impulse control.

> The condition affects 6.4 million children in the United States.

> The most common treatments recommended by doctors are stimulant and antidepressant medications.

> CBD and CBD-dominant cannabis cultivars may restore natural balance.

Attention-deficit hyperactivity disorder, or ADHD, is more than just an inability to sit still for a period of time. The lack of focus and patience, the restlessness, and the failure to cope with stress can have a huge impact on a person's life. Everyday chores such as doing schoolwork or driving a car can become herculean tasks when your brain is constantly detouring you away from what you are trying to do.

Stimulant and antidepressant treatments, which are the standard of care in the conventional medical community, often come with undesirable side effects. CBD offers an alternative. Its ability to soothe the nervous system and bring balance to the body is giving hope to those with ADHD.

Inside ADHD

ADHD is the preferred medical term for what was once called ADD. Although you probably have a good mental picture of what ADHD looks like, the term actually encompasses three branches of the disorder, each of which includes a spectrum of symptoms.

> **INATTENTIVE OR PREDOMINANTLY INATTENTIVE ADHD,** characterized by distracted behavior and carelessness, is often mistaken for anxiety. It is more difficult to diagnose because the symptoms are subtler than in its boisterous counterpart.

> **HYPERACTIVE-IMPULSIVE ADHD** is the type most people imagine when they hear "ADHD." Fidgeting, incessant talking, impatience, and struggling to follow directions are its hallmarks.

> **COMBINATION ADHD** is exactly what it sounds like—something in between the two.

CAUSES

Scientists are still trying to understand what causes ADHD, but they believe the following are factors:

> **FAMILY HISTORY.** Having blood relatives with ADHD, or even another mental health disorder, can put a person at risk.

A Real Problem

Nearly 10 percent of children in the United States have been diagnosed with ADHD, and the challenges they face in life are no joke. Kids with ADHD can struggle with:

> Poor performance in school

> Poor physical and mental health

> Poor self-image

And as they grow up, the stakes get higher. Teens and adults with ADHD can struggle with:

> Substance abuse

> Trouble with the law

> Unstable relationships

> Unemployment

> Car accidents

> Suicidal tendencies

Finding ways to cope with ADHD is essential to living a full and happy life.

> **ENVIRONMENT.** Researchers believe that early exposure to lead and other toxins can be correlated to ADHD symptoms.

> **DEVELOPMENTAL ISSUES.** Because the central nervous system plays a part, anything that affects a child's development in utero, such as the mother smoking, drinking, using pharmaceuticals and other drugs, or being exposed to toxins, can lead to ADHD.

SYMPTOMS

Hyperactivity is the hallmark symptom of ADHD; however, some equally detrimental symptoms can be so subtle that they are missed entirely. You may think someone is just a daydreamer or bad with details when he or she is actually in a daily battle with challenges such as:

> Impulsive behavior

> Disorganization

> Inability to focus or prioritize

> Poor multitasking and time-management skills

> Restlessness and impatience

> Inability to cope with stress

> Lack of follow-through

> Overall executive-functioning challenges

People who have gone through life undiagnosed may be unaware that their restlessness and difficulty concentrating are signs of ADHD. They have learned to cope with their "normal."

Who Is at Risk?

ADHD primarily affects children, especially those with a family history of developmental issues. Although the average child is not diagnosed until the age of seven, symptoms can appear in children as young as three years old. In addition:

> Boys are three times as likely as girls to be diagnosed with the disorder.

> Children living below double the federal poverty level are at higher risk.

> Children in English-speaking households are four times as likely to develop ADHD.

Symptoms tend to abate as people age, but roughly 4 percent of the adult population continues to live with diagnosed ADHD. Diagnoses of ADHD are on the rise.

The CBD Answer

There has been a 42 percent increase in ADHD diagnoses in the last eight years, which makes it seem like we are missing something that could bring about change. One hypothesis is that the previously unstudied endocannabinoid system may be to blame for ADHD, in which case, upregulating the endocannabinoid system with a CBD supplement may help correct the problem. But even if CBD does not turn out to be an end-all solution, cannabinoids still show great potential for ameliorating symptoms of the disorder—restlessness, insomnia, and impulsivity. Either way, CBD is a promising alternative to pharmaceuticals.

HOW TO USE IT

Because this condition mostly affects children, the best way to offer a CBD supplement for ADHD is with a tincture or gel cap. The amount to take really depends on the child and can vary even within the same child from day to day. As a general rule, start with a low dose two to three times per day. Using tinctures for children and for ADHD may be preferable, because you can easily change the dose to respond to behavioral and other changes.

Considering Edibles?

As a registered dietitian-nutritionist, I am not a fan of CBD-infused gummies and most infused chocolates for children.

> First, sweets are meant to be treats.

> Second, gummies and chocolates contain sugar, which can cause inflammation, and artificial ingredients such as flavors and colors, which can trigger hyperactive symptoms. (There are, however, a few infused-chocolate companies that make products with clean ingredients.)

Several decades ago, Dr. Ben Feingold theorized that certain added sugars and artificial ingredients triggered hyperactive behaviors. In fact, learning about the Feingold Diet was my introduction to the relationship between food and mood, and is one of the reasons I decided to study nutrition. My daughter Isabella (to whom this book is dedicated) brought me back full circle to the Feingold Diet. Funny how children can be our best teachers.

WHY IT WORKS

One theory is that ADHD is a manifestation of a clinical endocannabi-noid deficiency. (For a deeper discussion of clinical endocannabinoid deficiency, see pages 21–22.) Cannabinoids, including CBD, interact with the brain's production of dopamine, a neurotransmitter, so cannabis may alleviate ADHD by increasing dopamine levels. This is the same thing that stimulants do, but the mechanism of action and the side effects are different. The ADHD pharmaceuticals interfere with the dopamine pathway and come with a host of negative side effects. In addition to the potential benefits of cannabinoids in alleviating ADHD, this herbal supplement has proven to be valuable in relieving sleepless-ness and anxiety, both of which are symptoms of ADHD.

CBD VERSUS OTHER TREATMENTS

According to the Children and Adults with Attention-Deficit/Hyperactivity Disorder organization, ADHD costs Americans from $142 billion to $266 billion per year. Prescription drugs do not work for everyone and can have serious side effects, including insomnia, loss of appetite, and suicidal ideation. Sometimes people abuse their stimulant and antidepressant meds, leading to dependency. Not only can CBD modulate dopamine, but it can also address all of these side effects, making it a smart alternative therapy.

Natural Partners for CBD

Individuals with ADHD can use multiple techniques and lifestyle habits to help them manage. Here are a few:

> **GET SOME SLEEP.** Sleeplessness is a side effect of the disorder, especially for those suffering from the hyperactive-impulsive variety. Sleep in a cool, dark room without any electronics—that means no mobile phones. Get an old-school alarm clock!

> **AVOID TOXINS.** Environmental toxins, such as glyphosate and mercury, may exacerbate ADHD.

Making Connections

Exploring symptoms related to ADHD may be helpful. You can learn more in the chapters Anxiety Disorders (page 73) and Insomnia (page 161).

The Truth about Adult ADHD

Research suggests that as many as 70 percent of children with ADHD continue to experience symptoms as adolescents, and up to 60 percent will continue to do so into adulthood, which represents about 4 percent of the adult population. The 4 percent reported only accounts for those who have sought treatment for their symptoms and received a diagnosis. Too often, people assume that ADHD is a childhood affliction they will grow out of later in life. The negative impact of ADHD on a person's career, relationships, and overall life makes it all the more important for adults to seek solutions.

> **CUT OUT ARTIFICIAL INGREDIENTS.** Dr. Ben Feingold theorized that artificial flavors and colors triggered hyperactivity in children. Why do we need these scary ingredients anyway? Nature does such a good job of producing tasty flavors and spectacular colors!

> **CHANGE WHAT YOU EAT.** Studies reinforce that the proteins gluten (found in certain grains and many processed foods) and casein (found in dairy products) can contribute to behaviors associated with ADHD.

> **TAKE A FISH OIL SUPPLEMENT.** Studies have shown that omega-3 fish oil supplements may reduce the behaviors associated with ADHD. Always select supplements that meet or exceed international pharmaceutical standards.

> **GET YOUR MINERALS.** Studies have shown that ADHD is linked to low levels of iron and zinc, so including foods rich in these minerals or adding them as supplements may be necessary.

> **BREATHE DEEPLY.** Meditation and breathing practices can help people with ADHD slow down and refocus by affecting the endocannabinoid system.

AUTISM SPECTRUM DISORDER

> ➤ Autism spectrum disorder, ASD, refers to a range of developmental disorders that affect an individual's functioning across multiple areas of life.

> ➤ ASD affects one in 59 children in the United States, totaling 3.5 million Americans.

> ➤ The emotional, behavioral, and social functions that are disrupted in ASD are modulated by the endocannabinoid system, which makes CBD a promising treatment option.

Imagine: You are listening to the radio when static creeps in and distorts the sound. The noise gets worse, blaring painfully. Then the sound stops altogether. Even though you know the music is still playing somewhere, you cannot hear it. That is how Lori Sealy, an adult with autism, describes her personal experience. ASD is a whole-body

Making Connections

Exploring symptoms related to ASD may be helpful. You can learn more in these chapters: Anxiety Disorders (page 73), Appetite Loss (page 79), Chronic Inflammation (page 108), Epilepsy (page 138), Irritable Bowel Syndrome (page 167), and Insomnia (page 161).

disorder that impairs individuals' integration with the world around them. Autism can turn social interactions and activities of daily living into major challenges. New studies and plenty of anecdotal evidence suggest that cannabis and CBD can help.

Inside Autism Spectrum Disorder

ASD includes several formerly separate disorders, including Asperger's syndrome, with symptoms ranging from mild to life-altering—which is why it is called a "spectrum disorder." Communication and social interaction are almost always a challenge for people with ASD. Therapies usually revolve around alleviating symptoms and developing coping mechanisms. Typical medications include anticonvulsants, antipsychotics, and antidepressants—all of which can have dangerous side effects, especially for children. CBD may be able to take the place of those medications. Integrated with a specific food plan, targeted supplements, and other approaches, it did just that for my daughter.

CAUSES

No one knows what causes ASD, and even children who start out reaching developmental milestones can suddenly regress and show signs of the condition. Scientists believe that both genetics and environmental factors, such as pollution, viral infections, and toxins, may play a role. With no known cause and such a broad range of effects, ASD can be challenging to treat.

A Real Problem

Although we tend to focus on *children* with ASD, those children eventually grow up and become highly vulnerable adult members of society.

> Roughly 35 percent of adults with ASD need 24-hour support.

> While 87 percent of autistic adults live with their parents, only 22 percent want to.

> A staggering 67 percent of autistic individuals are victims of abuse.

The need for treatment options extends beyond the hope for happier, healthier kids—it is a requirement for strong, independent adults.

SYMPTOMS

No medical test can diagnose autism spectrum disorder, so watching for the following symptoms, especially in children under two, is crucial:

> Anxiety

> Epilepsy, or seizure disorders

> Sleep-pattern disturbances and insomnia

> Chronic inflammation

> Appetite issues, including specific food preferences

> Gastrointestinal issues

> Intellectual disability

> Poor social skills and little interest in interacting with others

> Speech disorders, such as apraxia

> Poor communication skills, including difficulty with expressive and receptive language

> Loss of language skills, which is a hallmark of regressive autism

> Sensory integration disorder, including sensitivity to light, sound, touch, and textures

> Repetitive behaviors such as rocking, spinning, and hand flapping

> Lack of joint engagement, such as pointing to show something

> Lack of imagination, including inability to engage in make-believe play

> Behavioral issues, such as aggression and fixation

Because the severity of the disorder can vary greatly, no overview of symptoms can cover all traits entirely. Generally speaking, if your child is under the age of two and shows signs of developmental delay, seek the guidance of a healthcare practitioner who specializes in treating ASD as a whole-body disorder.

Who Is at Risk?

Although researchers have yet to determine an exact cause, they have noticed a few consistent risk factors, including:

> **FAMILY HISTORY.** Having a child with autism makes you more likely to have another child with the disorder.

- ➤ **GENDER.** Boys are four times as likely as girls to develop ASD.

- ➤ **OTHER DISORDERS.** Children with fragile X syndrome, tuberous sclerosis, and Rett syndrome all have an increased risk of having ASD.

- ➤ **TOXIC EXPOSURE.** Exposure to glyphosate and other chemicals and heavy metals, such as mercury, may increase the risk of ASD.

- ➤ **PREMATURE DELIVERY.** Babies born earlier than 26 weeks, which is considered extreme preterm delivery, have a higher risk of developing ASD.

The CBD Answer

The endocannabinoid system is responsible for mood, pain, sleep, appetite, pleasure, motor control, and memory—all of which are challenged by autism. Scientists believe that the endocannabinoid system is involved in the progression of ASD. While research is still ongoing, parents who have used cannabis and CBD sing its praises.

HOW TO USE IT

Tinctures are the preferred mode of administration for individuals with autism, for two reasons. One, the dose can be changed easily. Two, sometimes individuals with autism have difficulty swallowing

Top Complications of ASD

Whether the symptoms are mild or severe, a person with autism spectrum disorder may face unique challenges in life, including:

- ➤ Problems in school—both learning and behavioral
- ➤ Social isolation
- ➤ Lack of independence
- ➤ Difficulties with employment—both getting and keeping jobs
- ➤ Bullying
- ➤ Stress on family and caretakers, which magnifies stress for the individual with ASD

These complications make it all the more important to find treatment options that are free of side effects. This can mean the difference between living and existing for someone with ASD.

pills. In certain instances, CBD-infused edibles or teas are a good idea. The point is that you treat the individual, not the condition. Because people with ASD may not be able to communicate, starting with a low dose and monitoring its effects is especially important. It may take time to find that perfect dose.

WHY IT WORKS

Many people with ASD have increased sensitivity to sounds, smells, textures, and lights. This sensitivity is a diagnosis in itself, referred to as sensory processing disorder. CBD normalizes GABA signaling and helps the brain stop the sensory overload that leads to anxiety and impaired social interaction. CBD is also a well-known treatment for epilepsy, which affects about 20 percent of people with autism.

CBD VERSUS OTHER TREATMENTS

Not only is there no specific cure for autism, but there is also no standard medical treatment. Different interventions work for different people, depending on where they are on the spectrum and how the disorder affects them. Finding what works is all about trial and error. The medications that treat the symptoms of ASD (hyperactivity, anxiety, behavioral problems) can all have dangerous side effects that are not fully understood, especially in relation to children. (Learn more in the Attention-Deficit Hyperactivity Disorder chapter, page 92.) With its promising record, CBD is certainly a treatment option for autism spectrum disorder.

Natural Partners for CBD

Because food is a healing tool that nature has provided us, combined with the fact that many pharmaceuticals do not actually treat ASD and instead cause harm, nutrition is an optimal route to take, especially integrated with CBD. Seek the guidance of a healthcare practitioner competent in using food as medicine, and in using cannabis for ASD. In addition to taking a CBD supplement, individuals with ASD may want to:

> ➤ **OPTIMIZE NUTRITION.** Food and nutrition can be potent modifiers for individuals with autism. Following an anti-inflammatory food plan with restorative fats and high-quality protein, along with eliminating gluten, casein, and artificial

ingredients while adding targeted supplements, can be used to treat the gut–brain axis. (For further discussion of the gut–brain connection, see page 74.)

> **MAINTAIN GUT HEALTH.** More and more, researchers are finding that having a healthy balance of bacteria is essential in overall wellness and for individuals with autism. Probiotics are a key part of the healing toolbox for individuals with autism.

> **DETOX.** Detoxification is a natural bodily process; however, individuals with autism typically have poor detoxification systems. Making these systems work optimally is a vital component of a personalized lifestyle plan for individuals with autism.

- Certain foods and herbs can be potent detoxifiers. Most are also considered anti-inflammatory.

- Water is the ultimate detoxifier: "The solution to pollution is dilution!"

- Sweating is one way that we detox, and this can be an issue for some individuals with ASD. A regular sauna may be an option.

CANCER

> ➤ Cancer causes your body's cells to divide and spread uncontrollably, destroying healthy tissue in the process.

> ➤ Each year, about 18 million people around the world discover they have one of hundreds of types of cancers.

> ➤ Cannabis with both CBD and THC, as well as other cannabinoids, can alleviate the side effects of cancer treatment.

Cancer invades so many lives. Whether you are one of the millions who battle this disease, or you love even one of those millions, cancer can be devastating. Incorporating cannabis with both CBD and THC may someday become an integral part of preventing or even combatting certain cancers. More research is needed to determine the efficacy of cannabis in cancer treatment. Until then, cannabis can help people fighting cancer by relieving the side effects of chemotherapy treatments.

Inside Cancer

Our cells are constantly changing: old ones die and new ones develop to replace them. But when cancer's at play, abnormal cells multiply uncontrollably. These extra cells can form tumors, which invade and wreak havoc on healthy tissue. They can also escape and spread through the lymph or blood to other parts of the body, which is a process called metastasis. With the odds of getting cancer now nearing 40 percent, we desperately need new ways to fight it.

CAUSES

Cancer is caused by changes to the genes that control how cells function. Any number of factors, however, can trigger those changes. Some of these factors include family history, exposure to toxins, sun exposure, consumption of carcinogenic foods, and smoking.

SYMPTOMS

With hundreds of types of cancers and multiple triggers, symptoms vary. General signs of the disease may include:

- ➤ Fatigue
- ➤ Unexplained changes in weight, skin, and bathroom habits
- ➤ Trouble breathing
- ➤ Difficulty swallowing
- ➤ Indigestion or discomfort after eating
- ➤ Unexplained muscle or joint pain, fever, bleeding, or bruising

Who Is at Risk?

Even individuals who lead clean lifestyles have developed cancer. Here are some factors that may increase your chances:

- ➤ **FAMILY HISTORY.** If cancer is a common branch in your family tree, your family members may be passing along a particular genetic mutation that increases risk.
- ➤ **GENDER.** Studies have shown that men are more likely than women to get cancer and less likely to survive it.
- ➤ **AGE.** Although cancer can crop up at any age, it usually takes time to develop. That is why people tend to be over the age of 50 when diagnosed.
- ➤ **HABITS.** Smoking, excessive drinking, eating an inflammatory diet, excessive sun tanning, and taking in toxins through foods, beverages, and other products can lead to certain cancers.
- ➤ **ENVIRONMENT.** Although people are becoming more conscious of greening up their environment, exposure to toxins is likely a major factor.
- ➤ **STRESS.** Along with lack of social support and depression, stress has been implicated as a risk factor for cancer progression.

The CBD Answer

When something as serious as cancer strikes, you throw everything you have at it. That may include conventional medical treatments as well as holistic options. Because cannabis and cannabinoids help to relieve pain, nausea, anxiety, and insomnia—all side effects of chemotherapy treatments—they can be a valuable holistic adjunct to conventional treatment. Marinol is a synthetic THC drug that has been approved for use in appetite stimulation in cancer for decades.

HOW TO USE IT

For relief of nausea and vomiting during cancer treatments, a CBD suppository or mouth spray may offer immediate relief. As usual with cannabis, start low and go slow. And remember that most of the studies and anecdotal evidence about cancer and cannabis are about cannabis with both CBD and THC.

WHY IT WORKS

Cannabis works for cancer patients by treating:

> **PAIN.** CBD reduces pain-causing inflammation and irritation.

> **NAUSEA AND VOMITING.** Cannabis acts on specific central nervous system receptors to decrease feelings of nausea, lessen the occurrence of vomiting, and increase appetite.

> **ANXIETY.** CBD boosts serotonin levels to quell anxiety and relieve insomnia.

CBD VERSUS OTHER TREATMENTS

Keep in mind that CBD alone is not an alternative to conventional treatment for cancer. Delaying chemo and radiation for early-stage solid tumors is not recommended in cases in which the probability of such appropriately timed mainstream treatments have demonstrated curative effects.

Making Connections

Exploring symptoms related to cancer and cancer treatments may be helpful. You can learn more in the chapters Anxiety Disorders (page 73) and Chronic Pain (page 113).

Natural Partners for CBD

With cancer prevalence increasing, it may seem like there is nothing you can do to avoid it, but integrating cannabis and CBD with other several lifestyle changes may help:

> **GO EASY ON THE ALCOHOL.** Try to limit intake to one glass just a few times a week or less.

> **MOVE YOUR BODY.** Completing at least 300 minutes of moderate exercise per week has been shown to help prevent a number of diseases, cancer included.

> **EAT AN ANTI-INFLAMMATORY FOOD PLAN.** Consuming detoxifying foods, dark leafy green, restorative fats, and high-quality protein is a crucial piece of the puzzle to prevent cancer and other chronic diseases. Cruciferous vegetables such as broccoli, cauliflower, bok choy, and Brussels sprouts are great detoxifiers because they contain sulfur compounds. .

> **PRACTICE STRESS-REDUCING TECHNIQUES.** Stress, anxiety, depression, and social isolation may play a role in the progression of cancer. Certainly, living with cancer can contribute to anxiety and depression. Do what resonates for you to relax—maybe join a support group, meditate, practice yoga, read, take a hike, use essential oils, or drink a cup of tea. Keep in mind that CBD also may help to reduce anxiety and depression.

A Real Problem

Cancer is the second leading cause of death worldwide, and the stats are startling:

> Every year, 18 million people are diagnosed with cancer and 9.6 million people die from it.

> Based on the growth of the aging population, 21.6 million new cancer cases and 13 million cancer deaths are predicted by the year 2030.

> More than one-third of cancer cases are preventable, and another third can be cured with early diagnosis and treatment.

With already promising results, there has never been a better time for scientists to look into how cannabis and cannabinoids, such as CBD, may help prevent and treat this tough disease.

CHRONIC INFLAMMATION

> ➤ Chronic inflammation contributes to the majority of chronic diseases, including chronic fatigue, irritable bowel syndrome, fibromyalgia, and neurodegenerative disease.

> ➤ Inflammation plays a major role in autoimmune diseases.

> ➤ One of the hallmarks of CBD is its ability to modulate inflammation.

Everyone experiences *acute* inflammation—you smack your knee into the table and a painful red lump appears. That sore spot is your immune system working to protect and heal your body. Without acute inflammation, infections and wounds would go unchecked, so a little bit of inflammation is a good thing. What we are talking about here is *chronic* inflammation, which is not a good thing! It can occur when your body is attempting to fight an infection but is losing the battle, such as is frequently the case with Lyme disease. The good news is that CBD is a potent anti-inflammatory ingredient that may reduce chronic inflammation.

Inside Chronic Inflammation

Chronic inflammation is both symptom and ailment, stemming from and leading to numerous conditions. If you have any of the following illnesses, chronic inflammation may be at play:

- Active hepatitis
- Allergies and hay fever
- Alzheimer's disease
- Asthma
- Autism spectrum disorder
- Cancer
- Depression
- Diabetes
- Heart disease
- Obesity
- Peptic ulcer
- Periodontitis
- Rheumatoid arthritis
- Sinusitis
- Stroke
- Tuberculosis
- Ulcerative colitis and Crohn's disease

CAUSES

In addition to appearing as a symptom of other illnesses, chronic inflammation can be caused by:

- **AN INFLAMMATORY DIET.** A diet that is high in foods that promote inflammation—including sugar, gluten, and fried foods—can contribute to chronic inflammation.

- **SENSITIVITY TO FOOD INGREDIENTS.** Sensitivities or intolerances to certain foods and ingredients can contribute to chronic inflammation.

- **EXCESS WEIGHT.** Fat cells, especially in the abdomen, release substances that trigger inflammation.

- **EXPOSURE TO TOXINS.** Toxins in personal, cleaning, building, and other products can contribute to inflammation.

A Real Problem

Chronic inflammation contributes to the vast majority of chronic disease in the United States. Check out the stats:

- Allergies: 50 million
- Alzheimer's disease: 6 million
- Asthma: 25 million
- Depression: 16 million
- Diabetes: 29 million
- Cancer: 15 million
- Heart disease: 28 million

Imagine how these numbers could drop if we had no processed foods and followed an anti-inflammatory food plan! Add CBD to the mix to supercharge the anti-inflammatory effect.

SYMPTOMS

Where there is smoke, there is fire. With chronic inflammation, you may experience:

> Overall body aches and pains, especially in the joints

> Anxiety and depression

> Change in sleep patterns or insomnia

> Fatigue or low energy

> Gastrointestinal issues, such as constipation, diarrhea, bloating, and leaky gut

> Skin rashes, such as eczema and psoriasis

> Worsening allergies, asthma, or excessive mucus production

Of course, chronic inflammation can itself be a symptom of these health conditions.

Who Is at Risk?

Chronic inflammation is the kind of condition that can affect absolutely anyone given the right mixture of circumstances. Many of us are exposed to possible triggers (see "Causes"). Lifestyle habits, especially related to food choices, affect the body's inflammatory response.

The CBD Answer

Not only can this cannabinoid quell chronic inflammation, but CBD may prevent other chronic conditions from surfacing. In conjunction with an anti-inflammatory food plan and targeted supplements, CBD may rid you of your chronic inflammation entirely.

HOW TO USE IT

Because chronic inflammation is systemic, you always want to use CBD internally. A daily oral supplement may be helpful. If pain is an issue, you may want to *additionally* use a targeted topical cream. Of course, do not select edibles containing inflammatory food ingredients. CBD may eventually eliminate your chronic inflammation to the point that you no longer need it for pain management and are simply taking it as part of your wellness routine. Work with a healthcare professional knowledgeable about integrating CBD with lifestyle changes. If you are taking medications, be sure to check with your prescribing doctor.

WHY IT WORKS

The mechanism is simple but powerful: CBD is known, first and foremost, as a potent anti-inflammatory. To go deeper into how this cannabinoid alleviates inflammation throughout the body, check out the full discussion beginning on page 19.

CBD VERSUS OTHER TREATMENTS

Chronic inflammation can have serious consequences, and so can its treatments. Non-steroidal anti-inflammatory drugs, or NSAIDs, such as naproxen and ibuprofen, are the go-to options in mainstream medicine, yet this drug class was never intended for long-term use. Overuse can cause stomach ulcers, worsen asthma, and even increase your risk of heart attack or stroke. The side effects of the other option, corticosteroids, can be even worse: osteoporosis, hypertension, diabetes, vulnerability to infection, and glaucoma. CBD, on the other hand, can be taken daily without dangerous side effects and may be even more effective at alleviating inflammation.

Natural Partners for CBD

Treating chronic inflammation stemming from lifestyle choices is a manageable task. You can integrate CBD with several lifestyle habits:

> **CUT OUT SUGAR.** Removing inflammatory foods—which includes anything sugary or fried or gluten-containing—is first and foremost in extinguishing chronic inflammation.

> **ADD IN INFLAMMATION-FIGHTING FOODS.** Food also can help to prevent and quell inflammation. Look to extra virgin olive oil, nuts, leafy greens, fatty fish, berries, and herbs.

The Truth about Obesity

Obesity is considered an epidemic in the United States, affecting more than 93 million adults. The extra fat can have serious repercussions. Chronic inflammation is just the tip of the iceberg. Obesity can also contribute to heart attacks, diabetes, and cancer—a few of the top causes of preventable death. And that is the key: *preventable*. Maintaining an optimal weight is important to keep chronic inflammation in check and to avoid chronic disease.

> **CONSIDER TARGETED SUPPLEMENTS.** Nutritional supplements, including fish oil, resveratrol, turmeric, and probiotics, can be part of an overall wellness plan to both treat and prevent inflammation.

> **GET OFF THE COUCH.** *Moderate* exercise or movement activities are key, because overdoing it can cause more inflammation than it relieves. Movement activities can trigger the production of your own endocannabinoids, which help to mitigate inflammation and, well, make you feel great. The boost is not from your endorphins—it is from your endocannabinoids!

> **REDUCE STRESS.** Attempting to live a low-stress life is vital to dealing with chronic inflammation. Practices such as meditation, deep breathing, and restorative yoga can help balance your endocannabinoid system. And do not forget sex with orgasm! Of course, it is the endocannabinoid system, producing endocannabinoids, that make you feel blissful.

CHRONIC PAIN

> ➤ Chronic pain may develop from a number of conditions and lead to complications such as depression and insomnia.

> ➤ As many as 50 million Americans experience chronic pain.

> ➤ The cannabis plant has been used to treat pain since ancient civilization.

> ➤ CBD can help relieve chronic pain—especially if it is caused by inflammatory or neuropathic routes—and treat its side effects by targeting multiple receptors in the body.

Believe it or not, a little pain is a good thing. It is your body telling you that something is wrong so you know you need to respond. Where the pain occurs typically lets you know where the problem is, and how bad the pain is tells you what to do next. Without those pain signals, a common condition such as appendicitis would be deadly every time. But chronic pain—pain that lasts for 12 weeks or more regardless of injury—is not informative. It is incredibly disruptive and depressing.

Inside Chronic Pain

Chronic pain is a serious medical condition that can affect absolutely anyone. Whether it is the result of an injury that does not heal, the symptom of another chronic condition, or a phantom imprint of pain once experienced, it can have a huge impact on the sufferer's life. And with the opioid crisis raging in the United States, it is a problem that needs a better solution—now! CBD may be an answer.

CAUSES

Causes of chronic pain include injury, illness, and repeated stress. As cut-and-dried as that sounds, the actual cause of chronic pain can be a tricky thing to uncover. Even when you have a specific cause, such as nerve damage resulting from an injury, the pain can outlast that injury and sometimes develop a psychological element.

SYMPTOMS

Symptoms of chronic pain depend on many factors, including cause, biological makeup, and pain tolerance. Someone with nerve pain due to multiple sclerosis will have completely different symptoms than someone whose pain stems from a knee injury suffered during a car crash. But the bottom line is that chronic pain is defined as *any* sort of pain that lasts for 12 weeks or longer.

Who Is at Risk?

Anyone can suffer from chronic pain, but you are more likely to develop the condition if you have one of the following risk factors.

> **INJURY.** Any sort of injury, whether major or minor, can result in chronic pain. Maybe the injury does not heal well, there is nerve damage, or you end up with phantom pain.

A Real Problem

Individuals with chronic pain are more likely to feel depressed, lose sleep and productivity, and experience strain on relationships and finances. That is very bad news considering that:

> Comprehensive treatment with painkillers helps only 58 percent of individuals, and with serious side effects, including addiction.

> Chronic pain costs the United States as much as $635 billion per year in both healthcare and lost productivity.

Finding a treatment plan that can work long term is essential to being able to function day to day. CBD can succeed where other treatments fail because this cannabinoid can be both effective and well tolerated in treating chronic pain over time.

- > **ILLNESS.** Some conditions, such as arthritis and fibromyalgia, go hand-in-hand with chronic pain.

- > **SURGERY.** Anytime a doctor cuts into your body you are at risk of developing chronic pain.

- > **GENDER.** Women are more likely to experience chronic pain than men, especially migraines and face and jaw pain.

- > **WEIGHT.** Those who are overweight put more stress on their bodies, which can result in persistent pain.

The CBD Answer

Chronic pain is a condition that differs from person to person, experience to experience. CBD has demonstrated effectiveness in inflammatory and neuropathic pain. Keep in mind, however, that CBD has less of an effect on the central nervous system than cannabis with THC. As a neuroprotective and anti-inflammatory, CBD ameliorates the *cause* of the pain, not actually the pain itself. That means that results are not necessarily immediate. As a general rule, CBD can take at minimum several weeks to decrease underlying inflammation and several months to reduce neuropathy. In addition to diminishing the underlying cause of pain, CBD can help with accompanying conditions such as insomnia, nausea, and depression. Lower back pain is the most common reason for the use of cannabis with THC or CBD to treat pain.

HOW TO USE IT

How you treat chronic pain with CBD will depend on where and how you feel the pain. Most chronic pain conditions are best treated by

Top Areas Affected by Chronic Pain

Most individuals experience pain in a specific area of the body or related to a specific injury or surgery. The most common complaints are:

> Lower back pain
> Joint pain
> Headache
> Nerve pain

> Post-traumatic pain
> Postsurgical pain
> Cancer-related pain

layering CBD formats. Using a patch, an oral tincture, and a topical product over the course of the day may be helpful. If you are taking any other medication, be sure to consult your prescribing healthcare practitioner. **NOTE:** If your state allows it, using a cannabis product with THC can be even more helpful in the treatment of chronic pain.

WHY IT WORKS

CBD can reduce or sometimes eliminate pain by reducing inflammation, which is the underlying cause of the pain. This cannabinoid has been shown to bind to receptors that mediate pain perception, inflammation, and body temperature.

CBD VERSUS OTHER TREATMENTS

Conventional treatment for chronic pain has relied on non-steroidal anti-inflammatories, or NSAIDS, such as ibuprofen and naproxen, and opioids for severe pain. Certainly, the opioid epidemic has revealed that overprescribing painkillers is harmful. CBD, on the other hand, can offer pain relief without the side effects of NSAIDS or opioids.

Natural Partners for CBD

With opioid misuse at crisis level, it is more important than ever to find safe and effective pain remedies. Here are a few that you can try, integrated with your CBD supplement:

> ➤ **MOVE YOUR BODY.** Movement activities, such as restorative yoga, walking, tai chi, and stretching, are excellent ways to combat chronic pain.

> ➤ **GET A MASSAGE.** Do you really need an excuse to have a spa day? Not only do holistic therapies such as massage, acupressure, and acupuncture relieve pain, but they also release

Making Connections

Exploring health conditions related to chronic pain and common pain treatments may be helpful. You can learn more in these chapters: Addiction to Substances (page 62), Depression (page 122), Insomnia (page 161), and Nausea (page 190). If you know the cause of your pain (such as arthritis or fibromyalgia), be sure to check out that condition chapter as well.

The Truth about Opioid Addiction

Health and Human Services officially declared the opioid epidemic a public health emergency in 2017, thanks to the following 2016 stats:

> A shocking 11.5 million people misused prescription opioids.

> Every day, 116 people died—that is 42,249 for the year—from opioid-related drug overdoses.

> The economic cost of the opioid crisis totaled $504 billion.

Opioids are incredibly addictive. At the same time, this class of painkillers is misused because the drugs fail to relieve chronic pain. The result: individuals prescribed opioids take more meds in the hope of finding relief, leading to overdose.

---

endocannabinoids, which are literally bliss molecules. Look for practitioners who have experience working with chronic pain.

> **GET SOME FEEDBACK.** Biofeedback is a therapeutic technique that uses electrical sensors to help you learn how to relax your body and control your pain.

CONTACT DERMATITIS

> ➤ Contact dermatitis is the technical term for any skin inflammation caused by contact with a substance.

> ➤ The condition is common and almost unavoidable, so easy treatment options are essential.

> ➤ One of CBD's greatest claims to fame is that it calms all kinds of inflammation, including contact dermatitis.

We are encouraged to try new things, but sometimes those things do not agree with us. If they are foods or beauty products, you may find yourself with a case of contact dermatitis. Almost everyone has experienced this kind of reaction. Taking a preventive CBD supplement or applying a CBD-infused cream may take the sting out of common causes of contact dermatitis, such as poison ivy.

Inside Dermatitis

Contact dermatitis is simply skin inflammation caused by coming into contact with something that puts your inflammatory system on alert. Your skin's inflammatory response to this substance, which it sees as an invader, is a red, itchy rash, or hives. Because we come in contact with potential allergens every day, almost every person on earth has experienced it. But it is as treatable as it is common.

CAUSES

Contact dermatitis pops up when your immune system reacts to an irritant or allergen touching your skin. There are technically two types:

- ➤ **IRRITANT CONTACT DERMATITIS.** This kind of flare-up happens when irritants (think: rubbing alcohol or bleach) damage your skin's protective outer layer.

- ➤ **ALLERGIC CONTACT DERMATITIS.** Whether you touch it or eat it, an allergen can cause an immune reaction in your skin. For example, if your body believes that shrimp is an allergen, your throat may not close up, but you may experience a bad case of hives.

SYMPTOMS

You will definitely know contact dermatitis when you see it. It can cause:

- ➤ A red rash
- ➤ Itching
- ➤ Hives
- ➤ Tenderness
- ➤ Swelling
- ➤ Burning
- ➤ Dry, flaking skin
- ➤ Bumps and blisters, sometimes oozing

Note: Contact dermatitis is different from a skin infection. If you think your skin is infected, see a doctor as soon as possible.

Who Is at Risk?

Everyone is at risk for contact dermatitis, but working in certain professions can increase your risk by increasing your exposure to potential allergens. Vulnerable workers include:

- ➤ Medical and dental employees
- ➤ Metalworkers and construction workers
- ➤ Hair stylists and cosmetologists
- ➤ Dentists
- ➤ Mechanics
- ➤ Dry cleaners
- ➤ House cleaners—both inside and out
- ➤ Gardeners
- ➤ Artists
- ➤ Restaurant workers
- ➤ Plumbers

The CBD Answer

CBD was made for fighting inflammation, which makes it a good solution for sensitive or aggravated skin. Add to that its antioxidant properties and you will find that a little CBD can go a long way in treating the rashes, bumps, and flakes associated with skin irritation.

HOW TO USE IT

The best way to use CBD to relieve skin irritation is by applying an oil, salve, cream, lotion, or balm directly to the affected area. If you tend to be sensitive to personal products, avoid those with added fragrances and oils. Refer to the Environmental Working Group website (ewg.org) about toxins in products and how to evaluate them. The addition of essential oils and other soothing ingredients may be welcome.

WHY IT WORKS

Inflammation is your immune system's response to what it thinks is harmful. CBD targets receptors in the skin, which is the largest organ in the body, to calm and balance it. While CBD's anti-inflammatory properties reduce redness and irritation, its antioxidant properties help restore your skin's protective barrier.

CBD VERSUS OTHER TREATMENTS

Treating contact dermatitis in conventional medicine usually involves steroid creams and/or oral steroids and antihistamines, which can have serious side effects, especially when used long term. Unlike these medications, CBD has been shown to reduce inflammation and restores skin's protective barrier naturally, by bolstering and balancing the immune system.

The Truth about Patch Testing

If you are unsure what caused a reaction, your doctor may recommend a patch test, in which he or she applies small patches of known allergens to your body. This is a safe and controlled way to discover any oddly specific allergies, such as goat hair or mown grass. This method can also come in handy at home. If you are not sure how you are going to react to something such as a beauty product, test a very small amount on an out-of-the-way area of skin before applying it fully according to its directions.

Natural Partners for CBD

The best way to treat contact dermatitis is to stop it before it happens. A CBD supplement taken orally may help, and so can these measures:

> **PROTECT YOUR SKIN.** Sensitive to metals? Iron fabric patches over the insides of metal fasteners on your clothing. Going for a hike? Pick up a poison-ivy barrier cream. Working with harsh cleansers? Replace them with nontoxic ones and invest in a good pair of latex-free gloves.

> **WASH UP.** If you come into contact with something you know will irritate your skin, wash the area thoroughly with warm water and a mild, fragrance-free soap and rinse completely. Then wash your clothes or anything else that may have been exposed.

> **SLATHER TOXIN-FREE LOTION.** Moisturizing regularly and well can help restore and maintain your skin's natural protective barrier, which means fewer flare-ups. Refer to Environmental Working Group's website (ewg.org) for more information about selecting products.

DEPRESSION

> Depression is a mood disorder that produces not only emotional symptoms such as pervasive sadness but also physical symptoms such as aches and pains.

> The condition affects 16.2 million Americans and roughly 300 million people worldwide.

> Researchers believe that CBD may offer an alternative to anti-depressant pharmaceuticals.

Feeling a little down in the dumps is a normal reaction to negative life experiences. But depression is more than just a reaction—it is more than disappointment or grief. It is the absence of joy, a sense of hopelessness, and an inability to concentrate or make decisions. It can rob sufferers of relationships, careers, and happy, productive lives. While proper medical care for this serious mental health condition is a must, researchers believe that CBD may also be able to help

Inside Depression

With numerous possible risk factors, depression can afflict anyone at any time. The condition turns simple, everyday tasks into arduous efforts by making sufferers feel overwhelmingly sad, listless, and unfocused. At its worst, depression can cause feelings of worthlessness and hopelessness that lead to suicidal thoughts. But the good news is that depression can be treated by integrating CBD with holistic approaches, including mental health counseling, meditation, and lifestyle changes around food and nutrition.

CAUSES

Scientists know that there are biological and neurological factors, and that genetics and gender play a role. Other possible causes include:

- Low self-esteem
- Substance abuse
- Physical or sexual abuse
- Chronic illness
- Certain prescription medications
- Biochemical issues such as nutrient deficiencies, inflammation, and hormonal imbalances

New studies show that in some cases depression may be caused by an underlying issue in the endocannabinoid system, which makes CBD a promising treatment to try.

SYMPTOMS

When it comes to mood disorders, sufferers really have two sets of symptoms—the emotional and the physical. Emotional symptoms may include:

- Sadness
- Emptiness
- Excessive irritability
- Anxiety
- Restlessness
- Loss of interest in formerly happy pursuits
- Low self-esteem or feelings of guilt
- Focusing on what went wrong
- Suicidal thoughts

Physical symptoms may feel similar to the flu:

- Sleeping too much or not enough
- Fatigue
- Change in appetite
- Change in weight
- Difficulty concentrating or making decisions
- Unexplained aches and pains

Who Is at Risk?

Depression can strike anyone at any time, but a few factors can make someone more susceptible:

> **BRAIN CHEMISTRY.** New research suggests that depression may be the result of malfunctioning neurotransmitters.

> **FAMILY HISTORY.** There may be a genetic component to depression, which means that having a family member with the condition increases your odds. It is important to note, however, that the field of study called *epigenetics* has found that we can change how a gene is expressed through lifestyle modification.

> **GENDER.** Women are much more likely to suffer from depression, possibly because of hormone fluctuations that occur throughout the life cycle, including premenstrual syndrome, menopause, and childbirth.

The CBD Answer

Studies have shown that CBD restores balance in the same way as selective serotonin reuptake inhibitors, or SSRIs, but without their dangerous side effects.

HOW TO USE IT

Because depression is a pervasive condition, taking CBD regularly is key. You want to build it up and maintain its level in your system with various delivery systems. For flare-ups, you may want to consider a more direct and timely delivery method such as vaping. (For more

---

The Truth about Depression

American society has placed a heavy stigma on depression as weakness or invention. People misunderstand and minimize depression, treating this serious condition like nothing more than a bad mood. They expect sufferers to just snap out of it using their own willpower. Although it is treatable, battling depression requires a lot more than willpower. Belittling its effects has stopped sufferers from seeking the care they desperately need. Depression deserves the same respect and attention afforded to chronic diseases such as heart disease and diabetes.

---

information on vaping, see page 36.) If you are taking medication for depression, check with your prescribing practitioner about any interactions with CBD.

WHY IT WORKS

Basically, CBD works in the same way that antidepressants do. As with SSRI medications, CBD redirects serotonin and dopamine—dubbed the happiness and motivation molecules, respectively—to the synaptic space, which boosts your mood. It also helps the hippocampus—the part of the brain responsible for memory and cognition—to create neurons, which can relieve anxiety and depression. The neurotransmitter GABA, which is responsible for modulating sensory overload, can be dysregulated in depression. CBD appears to modify a receptor for GABA, which enhances the calming effect of this neurotransmitter.

CBD VERSUS OTHER TREATMENTS

Many depression sufferers avoid prescription medications because they say they do not feel like themselves on them. Many more believe in the stigma against depression and think that prescription meds

Top Types of Depression

You may suffer from a single bout of depression, or you could battle it for years. While depression takes many forms, these are the most common:

> **Persistent depression disorder.** This is a longer-lasting and more muted version of those feelings of sadness that lasts two or more years.

> **Bipolar disorder.** Also called manic depression, bipolar disorder sometimes, but not always, results in mood swings that range from high, hopeful energy to extreme hopelessness.

> **Seasonal depression.** Seasonal affective disorder is a kind of depression triggered by a lack of sunlight and typically lasts through autumn and winter.

> **Postpartum depression.** Up to 80 percent of new mothers experience some kind of depression after giving birth. Symptoms usually resolve in a week or two; when they last longer they can indicate a depressive disorder triggered by childbirth.

are unnecessary. CBD strikes the perfect balance, helping to relieve symptoms without major side effects and with no more fuss than a multivitamin.

Natural Partners for CBD

Depression is an uphill battle with or without prescription medications, which means you need to make lifestyle changes that support your well-being. Adding a CBD supplement to your daily to-do list may help. You should also:

> **SET MANAGEABLE GOALS.** Because sufferers often feel lethargic and unmotivated, it is good to set small goals that you know you will succeed at. Little things count, such as making your bed. The point is to keep yourself focused on the next task and feeling a sense of achievement.

> **GET INTO THE HABIT.** Depression can drain the structure from your life as you struggle to complete normal everyday tasks. Having a routine helps you get a handle on things and move from day to day productively.

> **EAT OPTIMALLY.** The food you eat affects brain health. In general, select anti-inflammatory foods such as vegetables, herbs, restorative fats, and high-quality proteins. Avoid pro-inflammatory foods such as sugar, gluten, and artificial ingredients.

A Real Problem

Most people have felt the effects of depression, whether personally or by watching helplessly as someone they love suffers. In fact:

> 11 percent of adolescents are diagnosed with a depressive disorder before turning 18;

> 6.9 percent of all adults in the country—a total of more than 16 million people—suffer from some form of depression; and

> 60 percent of individuals who die by suicide had a mood disorder such as depression.

The numbers prove that depression is a condition we need to take seriously.

Ask for Help

If someone you know is at risk of hurting him- or herself or others, call 911. Stay with that person, try to keep the individual calm, and remove any dangerous objects. If you or someone you know is considering suicide, call the National Suicide Prevention Lifeline at 800-273-TALK (8255).

> **MOVE YOUR BODY.** Movement activities can trigger the production of your own endocannabinoids, which help to boost your mood.

> **TALK IT OUT.** Whether you seek solace in a medical professional, a counselor, or a friend, having someone act as a sounding board can help you sort out the symptoms and emotions of depression and keep things from getting out of hand.

DIABETES

> Diabetes affects how your body uses glucose, or sugar, in your blood. Too much in your system can cause serious health problems.

> Diabetes is classified as type 1 and type 2 and affects 30 million Americans.

> CBD's immune-boosting and anti-inflammatory effects can help bring balance back to the body.

Millions of people are putting themselves at risk of developing type 2 diabetes. When bogged down by work or everyday obligations, they may grab fast-food takeout, consume sugary drinks and snacks, shun exercise, hang out on the couch glued to screens, and ignore their expanding waistlines—all of which can lead to type 2 diabetes. Integrating CBD with an anti-inflammatory food plan, targeted supplements, and movement activities can restore balance to your body's processes to possibly treat *and prevent* type 2 diabetes. Emerging research in animals has revealed that CBD and other cannabinoids may influence both the incidence and progression of type 1 diabetes.

Inside Diabetes

The two types of the disease have different causes. In type 1 diabetes, which is classified as an autoimmune disorder, the pancreas does not produce insulin. Type 1 diabetes always requires taking insulin. Individuals with type 2 diabetes typically become resistant to insulin. If they manage the condition well with specific lifestyle habits, individuals with type 2 may not need to take any meds and can even reverse their diabetes.

CAUSES

Both types of diabetes are caused by the body's not handling blood sugar properly, but there are key differences:

> **TYPE 1 DIABETES** is caused by the body's own immune system attacking and destroying the insulin-producing cells in the pancreas called islets of Langerhans.

> **TYPE 2 DIABETES** is caused by the body's becoming resistant to insulin. At first, your pancreas may work overtime to create more insulin, but eventually it may stop producing insulin.

> In both cases, individuals with diabetes cannot regulate blood sugar optimally, which can result in many other health conditions.

SYMPTOMS

While the severity of symptoms depends on the severity of the blood glucose imbalance, the symptoms themselves are shared by both types of diabetes when not managed:

> Abnormal hunger, called polyphagia

> Abnormal thirst, called polydipsia

> Frequent urination, called polyuria

> Unexplained weight loss

> Fatigue

> Irritability

> Blurry vision

> Slow healing

> Frequent infections

Promising Research about Brown Fat

You may have heard about brown fat—the mitochondria-packed fat cells that burn energy. Its cousin white fat, on the other hand, stores calories. Research has demonstrated that CBD may help convert white fat into brown fat, which in turn may help to balance insulin and blood sugar. More research about this exciting development is needed.

Who Is at Risk?

The following factors put you at greater risk of developing diabetes:

> **AGE.** Type 1 diabetes can crop up at any age, though most diagnoses occur at younger ages. Because type 2 diabetes is usually related to lifestyle habits, it is typically diagnosed after age 40.

> **FAMILY HISTORY.** People who have family members with type 1 diabetes are more likely to develop it.

> **WEIGHT.** Being overweight is the number-one risk factor for developing type 2 diabetes, though not all individuals with type 2 diabetes are overweight.

> **INACTIVITY.** Being physically active helps your body use up glucose and remain sensitive to insulin. Conversely, physical inactivity puts you at higher risk of developing type 2 diabetes. Essentially, your body needs to be active to metabolize glucose properly.

> **RACE.** Individuals who are African American, Hispanic American, American Indian, and Asian American are at a higher risk of type 2 diabetes. Things can go wrong—very wrong—when people change their food habits from those of their native lands

A Real Problem

Diabetes affects more than 30 million Americans, and 7 million of those do not even know they have it. That means they cannot prevent or treat the conditions that diabetes puts them at risk of developing:

> Heart disease

> Stroke

> High blood pressure

> Kidney disease

> Ketoacidosis

> Nerve damage, or neuropathy, which can lead to amputation

> Glaucoma, cataracts, other vision problems, and blindness

> Skin conditions

> Erectile dysfunction

Staying on top of blood sugar, early diagnosis, and optimal treatment can save lives, and CBD may be able to help.

to the Standard American Diet (referred to as SAD) of refined, processed, and fried foods, including fast food, salty snacks, packaged sweets, and soda, with few vegetables, fruits, nuts, and seeds, excessive dairy products and other animal products. And that is certainly *sad*.

> **GESTATIONAL DIABETES.** Developing diabetes during pregnancy, called gestational diabetes, increases the risk of developing type 2 diabetes later in life.

> **PCOS.** Women with PCOS, or polycystic ovarian syndrome, are at higher risk of developing type 2 diabetes.

> **CELIAC DISEASE.** There is a genetic link between type 1 diabetes and celiac disease, which increases risk.

The CBD Answer

Adding a CBD supplement may reduce the inflammation associated with type 2 diabetes while stabilizing blood sugar and acting as a neuroprotectant and anti-spasmodic to relieve gastrointestinal discomfort. Time will tell if CBD can positively impact type 1 diabetes sufficiently to change patient outcomes.

HOW TO USE IT

Diabetes—whether type 1 or type 2—is a serious condition and must be treated as such. If you have diabetes and you are taking medication, it is crucial for you to consult with a healthcare practitioner before incorporating CBD into your treatment plan. To prevent diabetes,

How Blood Sugar Works

Your blood sugar, or glucose, powers your body and brain. When you digest your food, the various types of sugars and carbohydrates in the food are broken down into glucose. The glucose gets absorbed in the stomach and small intestine and is released into the bloodstream. That is what happens if everything goes right. When you have type 1 diabetes, however, your immune system destroys your pancreas's ability to create insulin, which processes glucose. With type 2 diabetes, your cells do not respond well to insulin. The result in both cases is that glucose builds up in the bloodstream.

taking a daily CBD supplement along with making lifestyle modifications may be a good idea. Of course, if you select CBD-infused edibles, avoid those that contain inflammatory products such as sugar, gluten, and artificial ingredients.

WHY IT WORKS

Researchers have found multiple links between imbalances in the endocannabinoid system and both types of diabetes. Type 1 diabetes results from the immune system's attacking itself. Researchers believe that CBD may slow down damage to the pancreatic cells that are responsible for regulating insulin.

A powerful anti-inflammatory, CBD can head off type 2 diabetes by quelling inflammation and improving the body's ability to metabolize sugar. It can also help users maintain a healthy weight, which is key in both treating and preventing type 2 diabetes.

CBD VERSUS OTHER TREATMENTS

Diabetes medications focus on helping the body regulate blood sugar. They are often used in conjunction with lifestyle changes that also regulate blood sugar and reduce excess weight. The Diabetes Prevention Program found that people who exercised and lost weight reduced their risk of turning prediabetes into type 2 diabetes by 58 percent. At age 60 or older, that increases to a whopping 71 percent reduction.

You can get a blood test called hemoglobin A1C, which assesses your blood glucose levels over the previous three months, to determine if you have prediabetes. Making lifestyle modifications that involve food, nutrition, movement activities, and stress-reduction techniques is an important component of a program to prevent type 2 diabetes. Integrating CBD with lifestyle changes may help to optimize diabetes prevention and treatment.

The Truth about Tracking

If you have diabetes, keep up both short-term and longer-range checks of your blood glucose levels. Tracking your blood sugar levels with a home blood glucose monitor is an important part of your treatment plan. The hemoglobin A1C blood test gives a picture of your blood glucose levels over the previous three months.

Natural Partners for CBD

So much of preventing type 2 diabetes and treating either type of diabetes is about finding your balance. CBD can help with that, especially when integrated with these lifestyle changes:

> **ACHIEVE A HEALTHFUL BODY WEIGHT.** The best way to lose fat is to change what you eat. One option is to follow a modified ketogenic food plan with restorative fats, high-quality protein, limited carbohydrates, and no or very little sugar.

> **SELECT AN ANTI-INFLAMMATORY FOOD PLAN.** Foods that trigger inflammation, such as sugar, must be avoided and those that moderate inflammation, such as green, leafy vegetables and herbs, must be added. Selecting foods according to their glycemic index may be helpful as well. Work with a registered dietitian-nutritionist or certified diabetes educator, preferably one who has experience with CBD, to create a personalized food plan.

> **GET OFF THE COUCH.** One of the best ways to avoid type 2 diabetes is to move your body and maintain a healthful weight. You do not have to live at the gym. Gentle movement activities, such as walking or restorative yoga, may be exactly what your body needs.

> **FIND WAYS TO DE-STRESS.** Stress hormones produced by the adrenal glands can trigger a rise in blood glucose and stubborn belly fat. Individuals with excess weight around their midsections are at a higher risk for type 2 diabetes. Integrating stress-reduction techniques and activities is important.

> **CONSIDER TARGETED SUPPLEMENTS.** Nutritional supplements, such as cinnamon, chromium, alpha-lipoic acid, resveratrol, and berberine, can be helpful in the management of blood glucose. Consult with a nutrition professional who has expertise in integrative or functional medicine, as well as in cannabis.

ECZEMA

> Eczema, or atopic dermatitis, is a chronic condition that causes occasional flare-ups of red, itchy, sensitive skin.

> Ten percent of all Americans experience some form of the condition.

> CBD's anti-inflammatory effects work wonders on the immune system and can reduce flare-ups.

Most of us have come into contact with something that irritated our skin—that is called contact dermatitis (see page 118). But imagine that the resulting redness, itching, and discomfort were not just a fleeting reaction. With eczema, that irritation can show up at any time, thanks to an overactive immune system that sees everything as a threat. Without a cure, mainstream medicine offers individuals who

A Real Problem

Not only are the flaky red patches of skin associated with eczema irritating and itchy, but they can also be painful and embarrassing. In fact:

> Two-thirds of people with eczema say that the condition interferes with their work and household chores;

> 66 percent of adults say that eczema restricts what they eat and drink; and

> Nearly 40 percent of sufferers report turning down a job or educational opportunity because of the condition.

suffer from eczema corticosteroid and non-steroidal topical products to put on the skin—which at best provide only temporary relief and frequently do not work to treat the underlying condition. A CBD supplement, with its anti-inflammatory and antioxidant effects, may be able to make life a bit easier for people with eczema.

Inside Eczema

The term *eczema* comes from a Greek word that means "to boil over," which is an appropriate description of the condition. Roughly 31 million people in the United States—adults and kids alike—suffer from the red, raised, itchy skin caused by eczema. The condition most commonly crops up in children and can resolve as they grow up, but it can also result in a lifetime of uncomfortable flare-ups.

CAUSES

Eczema is caused by an overactive immune system. The system is triggered by what it thinks is a threat, such as a harsh soap, and produces inflammation to protect the body. Research has also shown that people with eczema have a mutation of the gene that creates filaggrin, a protein that helps our skin maintain its protective barrier. Without filaggrin, the skin is more susceptible to dryness and infection.

SYMPTOMS

Beyond dry, itchy skin other symptoms include:

> Red to brownish-gray or silver patches

> Small raised bumps that may ooze and crust

> Rough, scaly skin

> Raw, sensitive, swollen skin, especially where you have scratched

Who Is at Risk?

Because the condition is the result of a malfunctioning immune system, anyone can develop eczema. Consider it the luck of the draw. The only known risk factor for eczema in mainstream medicine is having a family history of the condition. Eczema often travels with asthma, especially in children. It is no coincidence that both eczema and asthma can be improved with CBD, considering that both conditions are autoimmune disorders with inflammation.

The CBD Answer

Eczema is an inflammatory condition caused by a malfunctioning immune system. Not only does CBD do its best work in balancing the immune system, but it also contains skin-soothing antioxidants.

HOW TO USE IT

Because eczema is both a chronic and a dermatological condition, you may want to layer your CBD by using it in two ways:

> ➤ For the inner workings, you can take a daily oral supplement or edible. Because eczema is an inflammatory condition, avoid inflammatory ingredients, such as sugar and artificial flavors and colorings, in your CBD product and in your food plan.

> ➤ To calm angry skin, you can apply a CBD-infused product in an olive or coconut oil base to the area as needed. Make sure that it is suitable for sensitive skin and does not contain any added fragrances. Consult the Environmental Working Group website (ewg.org) for more information about avoiding toxic ingredients.

WHY IT WORKS

CBD is a homerun for eczema treatment:

> ➤ First it tackles the immune system response that causes eczema by affecting CB2 receptors.

> ➤ Then it uses balancing and anti-anxiety effects to mitigate eczema triggers such as stress and hormone fluctuations.

> ➤ Finally, the compound's antioxidant powers help restore skin's natural protective barrier.

CBD VERSUS OTHER TREATMENTS

Hydrocortisone is the most common treatment for relieving itchy skin, but like all steroids, it can have side effects in large doses. CBD, on the other hand, can naturally calm the inflammation at the source and repair skin's protective barrier without any harmful side effects. Taking it as a daily supplement may help prevent flare-ups.

Natural Partners for CBD

An eczema flare-up is a good reminder to slow down and take care of yourself. Adding CBD to your routine can help restore and maintain wellness in eczema sufferers. Here are a few other things you can do:

> **MOISTURIZE EFFECTIVELY.** Because eczema is linked to a deficiency of the skin's natural protective barrier, keeping skin hydrated is key. But not all moisturizers are created equal. Look for thicker products, such as body butters, with the terms "barrier cream" or "skin repair" on the label and ceramides in the ingredients list. Avoid petroleum jelly, which is a toxic ingredient, and follow the recommendation for ingredients from Environmental Working Group. Apply after a shower.

> **MEDITATE.** A regular meditation practice can help reduce the stress and anxiety that may trigger eczema, and kick your endocannabinoid system into action. And, of course, CBD can be effective in alleviating anxiety. (You can learn more about CBD's ability to alleviate anxiety in the chapter beginning on page 73.)

> **BE GENTLE.** That means avoiding harsh body products, taking shorter showers and baths in warm—not hot—water, and patting skin dry with a super-soft towel.

> **HEAL YOURSELF FROM THE INSIDE OUT.** It can be helpful to follow an anti-inflammatory food plan that includes fatty fish, colorful fruits and vegetables, lacto-fermented vegetables, and detoxifying herbs and that eliminates gluten, dairy, soy, and artificial ingredients.

Top Eczema Triggers

If you have eczema, you can steer clear of your triggers. A few of the most common ones include:

> Dry skin

> Sweat

> Stress

> Cigarette smoke

> Allergens such as pollen and dust

> Soaps, detergents, and fragrances

> Antibacterial ointments

> Gluten, particularly for children who also have asthma

Your list may look a little different, so the key is to identify your specific triggers and avoid them.

EPILEPSY

> Epilepsy is a central nervous syndrome, or neurological, condition that causes seizures, which are disturbances in the brain's electrical activity.

> One in every 26 Americans will develop epilepsy at some point, with current estimates at 2.2 million in the United States.

> CBD has been demonstrated to help reduce seizures in certain cases.

Imagine you are going about your day—working at your desk, or maybe walking down an aisle at the grocery store—and the next thing you know, you are surrounded by people asking if you are okay. A seizure cuts off communication between the brain and the body. You are unconscious, but things are still happening. Maybe you just stare into space, or maybe you collapse. But one thing is for sure: you are not in control. Medications, surgery, devices, and specific food plans have been employed to treat epilepsy, yet seizures remain an issue for many individuals. CBD may offer an option for people with seizures.

Inside Epilepsy

Epilepsy is diagnosed when a person has had two or more unexplained seizures. Individuals may experience seizures once in a while or have several a day, depending on the particular type and severity of the condition. Seizures take a toll on the body and mind, and their unpredictability can lead to falls, injuries, drowning, and car accidents.

CAUSES

The brain communicates with the body by sending out electrical signals. Epilepsy causes random lightning storms in the brain: the signals misfire and communication comes to a halt. Unfortunately for the majority of individuals, there is no known cause. For others, common causes include:

> Genetics

> Head trauma

> Brain inflammation

> Brain conditions, such as tumors or strokes

> Infectious diseases, such as meningitis or AIDS

> Prenatal injury

> Developmental disorders, such as autism spectrum disorder

SYMPTOMS

Symptoms depend on the type of epilepsy. Common occurrences of seizures include:

> Sustained rhythmical jerking movements

> Weak or limp muscles

> Brief muscle or eyelid twitching

> Repeated automatic movements, such as lip smacking or chewing

> Changes in sensation, emotions, or cognition

Top Seizure Triggers

Seizure threshold describes the balance between excitatory and inhibitory signals in the brain, which affect an individual's susceptibility to *seizures*. Many people with seizures have a low seizure threshold, so that seizures can be triggered by:

> Sleep deprivation

> Stress

> Drugs or alcohol

> Hormonal changes

> Low blood sugar

> Excess caffeine

> Specific times of the day or night, particularly at dawn and dusk

> Disruption in gastrointestinal function

> Heart racing

> Change in body temperature

> Lack of movement

> Confusion

> Staring blankly

> Loss of consciousness or awareness

Who Is at Risk?

Although the cause of most types of epilepsy is unknown, a few factors can put you at higher risk for the condition:

> **AGE.** Epilepsy tends to affect children and older adults.

> **FAMILY HISTORY.** Having a family member with epilepsy increases your risk.

> **ATHLETES WHO PLAY CONTACT SPORTS.** Any sport that involves hitting, banging, or knocking players, such as football, hockey, and rugby, puts individuals at risk for traumatic brain injury, which increases the risk of seizures.

> **INDIVIDUALS WITH DEVELOPMENTAL DELAYS.** People diagnosed with autism spectrum disorder and other special needs frequently experience seizures.

A Real Problem

People who have been diagnosed with epilepsy often live in constant fear of an episode. A seizure can happen at any moment and may result in injury. Unfortunately, epilepsy is on the rise and difficult to treat:

> Every year, 150,000 Americans are diagnosed with epilepsy.

> Sixty percent of epilepsy cases have no known cause.

> One-third of individuals with epilepsy live with seizures because no treatment methods work.

That last statistic is heartbreaking and the reason we need more research into the benefits of CBD. It is already showing promise where other treatments have failed.

> **BRAIN INJURY OR INFECTION.** Anything that negatively affects the brain—head injury, stroke, and infection—can increase your risk of developing epilepsy.

The CBD Answer

Adding a CBD supplement may reduce the number of seizures and may relieve some of the stress that comes with the condition. Its neuro-protective and anti-inflammatory properties can make CBD a powerful addition to an epilepsy treatment plan. In fact, CBD has proven itself so successful in treating epilepsy that the first-ever CBD medication—Epidiolex—has been developed to treat a severe form of the condition.

HOW TO USE IT

If you have seizures, it is imperative to work with a healthcare practitioner skilled in treating seizures with CBD. Keep in mind that CBD is not a benign supplement in this population. Many individuals who have epilepsy take multiple medications, which makes it extremely important to monitor drug interactions with CBD. Seek the advice of a medical professional if you have seizures and are considering CBD.

WHY IT WORKS

Similar to some of the most common seizure medications, CBD blocks NMDA receptors, enhancing GABA receptors and stabilizing ion channels to reduce seizure activity. It also acts as an anti-inflammatory and neuroprotectant, which may help bring balance back to a misfiring brain. In addition, CBD's anti-anxiety effects may help with the stress of having an unpredictable seizure disorder.

CBD VERSUS OTHER TREATMENTS

A big problem with antiepileptics, or anti-seizure meds, is that they do not work for everyone. Some patients are resistant. One study found that the most treatment-resistant patients had 39 percent fewer seizures

Making Connections

Exploring health conditions related to seizures may be helpful. You can learn more in the chapters Anxiety Disorders (page 73) and Autism Spectrum Disorder (page 98) .

when taking CBD *in addition to their regular meds.* Epilepsy drugs can also come with side effects such as dizziness, drowsiness, skin rash, mental slowing, weight gain, kidney stones, metabolic acidosis, glaucoma, liver damage, colitis, and movement and behavioral disorders. Use of CBD by individuals with seizures can also have side effects, including sedation, diarrhea, vomiting, and insomnia. In some cases, seizures can be worsened and liver enzymes may become elevated, depending on other meds. Again, it is vital to check with your doctor if you have epilepsy and are taking medication before you embark on adding CBD to your treatment plan.

Natural Partners for CBD

Integrating CBD with other holistic modalities may help manage epilepsy for a better quality of life.

> **FOLLOW A SPECIFIC FOOD PLAN.** Studies have demonstrated that a ketogenic diet—high in fat, high in protein, and very low in carbohydrates—that encourages a metabolic process called ketosis can reduce and sometimes eliminate seizures. In some cases a Modified Atkins Diet, which is less restrictive than a ketogenic food plan, can be helpful. Treating blood glucose dysregulation may also be helpful for individuals with seizures. Working with a registered dietitian-nutritionist who has experience in treating seizures with food is recommended.

> **USE TARGETED SUPPLEMENTS.** Nutritional supplements, such as fish oil, L-carnitine, and B vitamins, can be incorporated into specific food plans to help manage seizures and overall health.

> **KEEP TABS ON TRIGGERS.** Identifying and avoiding triggering agents, such as alcohol, aspartame, monosodium glutamate, and salicylates, is crucial for some individuals with epilepsy. Not all triggers affect all people. Keeping a journal of your food habits, mood, activities, weather, stress level, and more can be helpful to figuring out which triggers affect you and improving your quality of life.

> **ADOPT A DOG.** Not only do animals help relieve the anxiety that comes with epilepsy, but specially trained seizure dogs can also respond to seizures by barking to alert caregivers, shielding sufferers from harm, and tripping an alarm.

FIBROMYALGIA

> Fibromyalgia is a debilitating condition whose primary symptoms include pain, insomnia, and fatigue.

> Roughly 10 million Americans suffer from fibromyalgia.

> Individuals who have fibromyalgia frequently experience migraines and gastrointestinal issues, possibly related to a clinical endocannabinoid deficiency.

> CBD may relieve the symptoms associated with this condition.

Not long ago, people suffering from widespread pain, fatigue, and general brain fog were told they were imagining the symptoms. Today, we know that fibromyalgia is real and devastating. Research suggests that cannabis with THC, as well as CBD, may be able to relieve the symptoms of fibromyalgia.

Inside Fibromyalgia

Researchers believe that fibromyalgia affects the way the brain processes pain signals, amplifying painful sensations. Sometimes the condition is the result of an injury or infection. Often, however, the pain accumulates over time with no known cause. Conventional treatment of fibromyalgia is about managing the symptoms and avoiding triggers.

CAUSES

The cause of fibromyalgia is unknown, but a few theories have been suggested:

> **GENETICS.** Having a family member with fibromyalgia seems to increase your risk. This factor suggests the possibility of a gene mutation that may get triggered to express itself.

> **PRIMARY CONDITIONS.** Fibromyalgia is sometimes secondary to illnesses such as rheumatoid arthritis and lupus.

> **PHYSICAL OR EMOTIONAL TRAUMA.** The stress of a severe injury or psychological event can sometimes trigger fibromyalgia.

> **CLINICAL ENDOCANNABINOID DEFICIENCY.** Neurologist and cannabis researcher Ethan Russo has suggested that some individuals do not produce sufficient endocannabinoids, which disrupts balance and homeostasis, possibly contributing to fibromyalgia and other medical conditions. (To learn more about clinical endocannabinoid deficiency, see the discussion that begins on page 21.)

SYMPTOMS

The main symptoms of fibromyalgia can be categorized:

> **PAIN ALL OVER.** The term "widespread pain" refers to pain that is experienced all over the entire body. In the case of fibromyalgia, it is usually a dull ache that lasts for more than three months, though it can be more severe.

> **FATIGUE.** Sometimes the pain keeps individuals from sleeping, and sometimes it wakes them up. Even when people with fibromyalgia get plenty of sleep, they still feel exhausted.

> **BRAIN FOG.** People with fibromyalgia have a difficult time paying attention and focusing on mental tasks.

Making Connections

Exploring symptoms related to fibromyalgia may be helpful. You can learn more in the Chronic Pain (page 113), Depression (page 122), and Insomnia (page 161) chapters.

Who Is at Risk?

No one knows what truly causes fibromyalgia, but researchers have noticed a few common threads:

> **GENDER.** The number-one risk factor for developing fibromyalgia is gender. Women account for a whopping 90 percent of cases.

> **FAMILY HISTORY.** Fibromyalgia seems to run in the family, so having a genetic link to someone with the disease can put you at risk.

> **OTHER CONDITIONS.** Suffering from lupus or arthritis can put you at greater risk of developing fibromyalgia.

The CBD Answer

The effectiveness of cannabis with THC for pain relief is well documented. Whole plant CBD has also demonstrated an ability to reduce pain—a hallmark symptom of fibromyalgia—as well as to alleviate anxiety, sleeplessness, and digestive issues. Many integrative cannabis clinicians believe that fibromyalgia is optimally treated by integrating cannabis with THC, even in small amounts.

HOW TO USE IT

A multi-pronged, or layered, approach may be warranted for fibromyalgia. That may mean taking a CBD oil or edible by mouth and also using a CBD-infused product topically on areas of pain. Sometimes, topical products with additional ingredients, such as relaxing essential oils or botanicals, can be helpful.

Top Fibromyalgia Triggers

Because fibromyalgia is a chronic condition, the most important aspect of treatment is learning to manage the disease and avoid triggers, such as:

> Stress

> Changes in weather

> Lack of sleep

> Injury

> Physical activity or inactivity

> Symptoms

WHY IT WORKS

One theory is that clinical endocannabinoid deficiency contributes to the development of fibromyalgia. The endocannabinoid system has been suggested to regulate the threshold for harmful stimuli, which is why cannabis works so well to relieve pain and restore quality of life. Another theory is that CBD works by desensitizing certain pain and heat receptors in the body, resulting in a decreased perception of pain by the nervous system. Additionally, the anti-inflammatory, antioxidant, and neuroprotective properties of CBD are also at play.

CBD VERSUS OTHER TREATMENTS

The pain of fibromyalgia may not be the only symptom, but it is usually the most pressing, which incites many to turn to over-the-counter pain relievers. When overused, these can cause ulcers and liver damage, but in the scheme of things that is preferable to getting hooked on opioids. Of course, because excessive opioid use can lead to adverse consequences, considering alternatives such as cannabis may be extremely beneficial to individuals with fibromyalgia.

Natural Partners for CBD

Self-care is one of the most important factors in treating fibromyalgia. Integrating CBD with other holistic practices can help you restore balance to your system:

> **EAT A PREBIOTIC AND PROBIOTIC FOOD PLAN.** A healthy microbiome—the community of microorganisms in your body—is vital for optimal health and plays a role in the gastrointestinal, neurological, and other systems. Select foods that provide prebiotics, such as artichokes, onions, garlic, and dandelion greens, plus probiotic foods, including lacto-fermented vegetables and kombucha. Consulting a nutritionist with experience in feeding the endocannabinoid system and treating fibromyalgia can be helpful.

> **CONSIDER TARGETED SUPPLEMENTS.** Fish oil, turmeric, ginger, boswellia, alpha-lipoic acid, and other nutritional supplements may be recommended. Be sure to work with a healthcare professional for specific recommendations.

> **TUNE IT OUT.** Practicing meditation may help to lower

A Real Problem

The pain of fibromyalgia is just one piece of the puzzle. Individuals with fibromyalgia are at higher risk of developing:

- Anxiety
- Arthritis
- Depression
- Digestive disorders
- Insomnia
- Migraine and tension headaches
- Temporomandibular joint (TMJ) disorders

---

stress—a major trigger—and to tune out the pain and anxiety fibromyalgia causes.

- **MOVE YOUR BODY.** Movement activities are essential to relieving fibromyalgia pain. Low-impact activities such as swimming and restorative yoga are particularly good choices.

- **TALK IT OUT.** Depression is a real concern when it comes to fibromyalgia. If you are feeling anxious or overwhelmed, find a mental health counselor who can help you cope.

- **GO FOR BODY TREATMENTS.** Both acupuncture and massage can be helpful in reducing the pain associated with fibromyalgia.

GLAUCOMA

> ➤ Glaucoma is a group of eye disorders that cause abnormally high intraocular pressure, which can damage the optic nerve and result in vision loss.

> ➤ Over 3 million people have glaucoma, and it is the leading cause of blindness in the United States.

> ➤ Small doses of THC, *not* CBD, have been shown to reduce intraocular pressure.

Every year, you go for an eye exam and sit at a little machine where you are told not to blink as you stare at a spot on a screen. You know what is about to happen—that little puff of air is coming straight for your eye. This is a test of your intraocular pressure; if it is too high, you could be at risk of glaucoma and irreversible vision loss. THC may offer hope to reduce the pressure and risk.

Inside Glaucoma

Glaucoma is the result of excessive pressure in your eye, causing damage to the optic nerve. Over time, you develop spots on your vision that can lead to blindness in one or both eyes. If you catch it early, you can take measures to reduce the pressure and prevent any more damage. But half of all people who have glaucoma do not know they have it, so vision tests are key.

CAUSES

Glaucoma is caused by damage to the optic nerve, which creates blind spots as it deteriorates. That nerve damage usually has something to do with elevated eye pressure, when fluid builds up on the eye rather than draining out through tissue.

SYMPTOMS

The scary thing about open-angle glaucoma, which is the most common kind, is that you do not notice symptoms until things have seriously deteriorated. At that point you will notice blind spots or tunnel vision. Symptoms of acute-angle glaucoma include:

- Severe headache
- Eye pain and redness
- Nausea
- Blurry vision
- Halos around lights

Who Is at Risk?

Glaucoma can start destroying your vision well before you have any idea it is happening, so it is a good idea to be aware of risk factors:

- **AGE.** Although anyone can develop glaucoma, people over the age of 60 are at higher risk.

- **RACE.** People who are black or Hispanic are more likely than whites to develop the disease.

- **FAMILY HISTORY.** You are at higher risk for the condition if you have a family member who has glaucoma.

- **OTHER CONDITIONS.** People who have diabetes, heart disease, high blood pressure, and sickle cell anemia have an increased risk of developing glaucoma.

A Real Problem

While glaucoma is a serious condition for everyone affected, it is especially worrisome for people of color:

- Black people are 15 times more likely to develop glaucoma.
- The disease strikes earlier and progresses faster in people of color.
- Blindness from glaucoma is six to eight times more common in black people than white people.

Early detection is imperative for people of color, so getting regular tests for glaucoma starting at age 35 is recommended.

Is Cannabis an Answer?

Studies have shown that cannabis with THC, not CBD, may help with glaucoma. Regardless, many medical marijuana doctors only recommend THC-containing cannabis in conjunction with glaucoma medication. *At this time, CBD is not recommended for glaucoma.*

HOW TO USE IT

CBD has not been found to relieve the intraocular eye pressure associated with glaucoma. For use of cannabis with THC to treat glaucoma, consult a practitioner in a state where medical marijuana is legal.

WHY IT MAY WORK

The endocannabinoid system plays a role in overall eye health because the retina, an integral part of the central nervous system, contains endocannabinoid receptors. Ocular CB1 receptors are directly involved in regulating intraocular pressure, meaning that cannabis with THC can have a localized effect on the retina and the optic nerve. Nearly a decade ago, the American Academy of Ophthalmology classified glaucoma as a neuro-degenerative disease.

Natural Partners for Prevention

With glaucoma, an ounce of prevention is worth a pound of cure. For possible glaucoma prevention, you can:

> **GET MOVING.** Movement activities that raise the pulse by just 20 to 25 percent may be helpful to lower intraocular pressure. One option that fits this range: taking a brisk walk for 20 minutes about four times weekly.

> **EAT EYE-LOVING FOODS.** To keep any sort of eye ailment at bay, make sure you eat an anti-inflammatory food plan, rich in dark, leafy greens, flavonoid-rich vegetables and fruits, and fish high in omega-3 fatty acids. You may also want to consider a nutritional supplement specifically formulated for eye health.

> **GO EASY ON THE COFFEE.** Drinking beverages high in caffeine has been shown to increase intraocular pressure in some cases, so decreasing caffeine intake may be a good idea.

HEART DISEASE

> Heart disease is caused by hardened blood vessels and plaque build-up—called atherosclerosis—that reduces the heart's ability to function and can lead to a heart attack.

> Heart disease is the leading cause of death for both men and women in the United States.

> CBD may alleviate the chronic inflammation associated with heart disease and may also lower blood pressure and minimize arrhythmias.

Everyone has made choices that negatively affect health, whether it be grabbing fast food or getting sucked into binge-watching. There can also be that ever-present black cloud of stress and anxiety. Poor lifestyle choices and a lack of stress-reduction techniques, possibly combined with a genetic predisposition, can lead to heart disease. Integrated with optimal wellness practices, CBD can support heart health by helping people to maintain a healthy weight, a regular heartbeat, normal blood pressure, and a balanced immune system.

Top Complications of Heart Disease

Heart disease can lead to:

> Heart failure

> Heart attack

> Stroke

> Aneurysm

> Peripheral artery disease

> Sudden cardiac arrest

Inside Heart Disease

Heart disease is the umbrella term for various health conditions, including cardiovascular disease, arrhythmias, congenital defects, cardiomyopathy, valvular heart disease, and heart infection. Heart disease is the number-one killer of all people in the United States.

CAUSES

The cause of heart disease varies by the type.

TYPE OF HEART DISEASE	CAUSE
Cardiovascular disease	Plaque buildup that reduces blood flow
Arrhythmia	Defects, high blood pressure, drug abuse, and stress, among others
Congenital defects	Appear as the heart develops and changes
Cardiomyopathy	Unknown, possibly reduced blood flow
Valvular heart disease	Rheumatic fever, infection, connective tissue disorder
Heart infection	Bacteria, virus, parasite

SYMPTOMS

The symptoms associated with the various forms of heart disease are many, including:

> Chest pain or pressure

> Shortness of breath

> Upper-body pain

> Racing heartbeat

> Unexplained swelling

> Lightheadedness

> Fatigue

> Fainting

Who Is at Risk?

The list of risk factors for heart disease includes:

> **AGE.** As you age, so does your heart muscle, which affects its ability to function well.

> **GENDER.** Men have a greater risk of heart disease, though women catch up after menopause and are less likely to survive a heart attack.

> **FAMILY HISTORY.** Having a family member with a heart condition increases your odds; however, your genes are not your destiny. You can modify your chances of developing heart disease by changing your lifestyle habits.

> **SMOKING.** The nicotine and carbon monoxide in cigarettes narrow and damage your arteries, increasing the chances of having a heart attack.

> **CANCER MEDS.** Certain chemotherapy drugs and radiation can affect your heart health.

> **AN INFLAMMATORY DIET.** Consuming foods that contribute to chronic inflammation can increase your risk of developing heart disease.

> **HIGH BLOOD PRESSURE.** High blood pressure, or hypertension, can cause thickening arteries and narrowed blood vessels, making it harder for blood to reach your heart.

> **BLOOD CHOLESTEROL LEVELS.** Elevated levels of very low-density lipoprotein fractions, low levels of high-density lipoproteins, and high triglycerides increase risk.

> **DIABETES.** Individuals who have diabetes are more likely to develop heart disease.

> **OBESITY.** Excess weight puts stress on your heart, making it work harder and wear out faster.

> **LACK OF MOVEMENT.** The heart is a muscle, which means it requires movement activities to stay healthy.

> **STRESS.** Excess stress can weaken arteries and add to the weight of other risk factors.

> **POOR HYGIENE.** Anything that puts you at risk of infections can increase your risk of heart disease.

The CBD Answer

Having a daily wellness routine that includes a heart-healthy food plan, incorporates movement activities, and reduces stress is imperative to prevent and treat heart disease. With its system-balancing, immune-supporting properties, CBD can be a helpful addition to that routine.

Making Connections

Exploring conditions related to heart disease may be helpful. You can learn more in the chapters Anxiety Disorders (page 73), Chronic Inflammation (page 108), and Diabetes (page 128) .

HOW TO USE IT

CBD may be appropriate in reducing risk of heart disease. If you are taking any meds, check with your prescribing doctor before using CBD to understand how it may interact with medications used to treat high blood cholesterol and high blood pressure, among other meds.

WHY IT WORKS

Researchers believe that CBD may help individuals with heart disease by attacking these heart disease–related health issues:

> **CHRONIC INFLAMMATION.** CBD's anti-inflammatory properties may keep the immune system from overreacting and causing more damage.

> **BLOOD PRESSURE.** Very preliminary research has demonstrated that a single large dose of CBD reduced resting blood pressure and the blood pressure response to physiological stress. More studies are needed.

> **ARRHYTHMIAS.** Studies conducted *in vivo* suggest that CBD works as an anti-arrhythmia and may improve recovery from stroke.

> **TISSUE-SPARING.** In animal studies, CBD appeared to reduce the area of the heart muscle that had been damaged.

Additionally, CBD may mitigate the anxiety experienced by individuals with heart disease.

A Real Problem

Only a small fraction of people know that chest pain is not the only symptom of a heart attack; others include nausea, upper-body and abdominal pain, sweating, and shortness of breath. This means that many individuals miss the warning signs that can save their lives. Consider:

> 28.1 million people have been diagnosed with heart disease in the United States;

> 735,000 have heart attacks each year; and

> 633,000 die from heart disease each year, which accounts for one of every four deaths.

Optimizing lifestyle choices and knowing the symptoms of a heart attack can help people avoid fatalities.

CBD VERSUS OTHER TREATMENTS

CBD cannot cure heart disease. This cannabinoid may reduce inflammation and oxidative stress and, in turn, reduce the risk of developing heart disease and prevent other consequences, such as heart failure. Integrated with lifestyle changes, CBD may increase your overall wellness and reduce risk of heart disease.

Natural Partners for CBD

Preventing and treating heart disease are both about living a more balanced life, which makes CBD a sensible addition to your wellness plan. Here are a few ways to find that balance:

> **EAT HEART-HEALTHFULLY.** The food we eat has a huge impact on our hearts. A food plan that includes an abundance of vegetables and fruits, fish, eggs, nuts, and restorative fats can have anti-inflammatory benefits. Keeping red meat intake occasional is also recommended for heart health.

> **MOVE YOUR BODY.** Regular movement activities help people to maintain weight, exercise the heart muscle, lower blood pressure, improve blood cholesterol, and regulate blood sugar.

> **CONSIDER TARGETED SUPPLEMENTS.** Several nutritional supplements are recommended for heart health, including omega-3 fatty acids, CoQ-10, magnesium, niacin, and L-ribose. Always check with a functional medicine nutritionist for your specific supplement recommendations.

> **MAKE TIME TO DE-STRESS.** Feeling stressed out all the time can take a heavy toll on your heart. Whether you turn to meditation or leisure reading, find ways to relax. Keep in mind that CBD also may help to reduce anxiety.

INFLAMMATORY BOWEL DISEASE

> ➤ Inflammatory bowel disease (IBD) is an autoimmune disease that causes chronic inflammation of the digestive tract, resulting in severe symptoms.

> ➤ Roughly 1.6 million people in the United States have IBD, and that number is growing.

> ➤ CBD's major claim to fame is its anti-inflammatory effect, which makes it an option for people with IBD.

Everyone experiences gastrointestinal issues once in a while. Inflammatory bowel disease, on the other hand, is on a whole different level from stomach upset. IBD typically has a profound impact on quality of life. Day-to-day symptoms are often exhausting, and many individuals with IBD need life-altering surgery. Studies show that CBD may be able to help with symptoms of IBD.

IBD versus IBS

It is important to recognize that inflammatory bowel disease and irritable bowel syndrome (IBS) are two different conditions, although there can be overlap in symptoms. IBD is a serious, chronic condition characterized by intestinal inflammation. IBS, on the other hand, is a less serious and more common disorder that affects muscle contractions. For more information on IBS, see page 167.

Inside IBD

IBD is an umbrella term for conditions caused by chronic inflammation in the digestive tract—namely Crohn's disease and ulcerative colitis. Crohn's describes inflammation that goes deep into the tissue of the digestive tract, while ulcerative colitis is characterized by inflammation and sores, or ulcers, in the colon and rectum. Both illnesses can cause severe diarrhea, abdominal pain, and fatigue.

CAUSES

Scientists believe that IBD is caused by a malfunctioning immune system that attacks cells in the digestive tract, leading to chronic inflammation that damages the area.

SYMPTOMS

Symptoms of IBD can be anywhere on the spectrum of mild to severe and usually include:

- Diarrhea
- Fever
- Fatigue
- Abdominal pain and cramping
- Bloody stool
- Loss of appetite
- Unexplained weight loss

Who Is at Risk?

The following factors can increase your chances of developing IBD:

- **ANCESTRY.** Being of Ashkenazi Jewish descent increases your risk of developing IBD, likely attributable to a genetic mutation.

- **AGE.** Although you can develop IBD at any age, you are more likely to see symptoms before turning 30.

- **RACE.** White people have the highest risk of developing IBD.

- **FAMILY HISTORY.** Having a family member who suffers from IBD increases your risk.

- **SMOKING.** A nicotine habit not only increases your risk of developing Crohn's but can also increase the severity of the disease.

- **MEDICATIONS.** Nonsteroidal anti-inflammatory drugs, such as ibuprofen and naproxen, can increase your risk of developing IBD and can worsen its symptoms.

> **LIFESTYLE.** Living in an industrialized nation increases your risk for IBD, suggesting that IBD is linked to lifestyle choices such as eating habits.

The CBD Answer

Cannabis with THC has been used to treat digestive disorders for centuries. In fact, IBD is a qualifying condition for a marijuana recommendation in many states with medical marijuana laws. For individuals who do not have access to medical marijuana, CBD can offer an option for treating ulcerative colitis and Crohn's because of its immune-supporting, anti-inflammatory properties.

HOW TO USE IT

The recommended way to use CBD for IBD is in a sublingual oil—meaning under the tongue. You can also use vaporizers for quick relief during a flare-up. Be sure to consult with a health professional about products, especially if you are taking medications.

WHY IT WORKS

Clinical endocannabinoid deficiency may be a contributing factor in the development of IBD. The gastrointestinal system is loaded with endocannabinoid receptors, which appear to become activated when

A Real Problem

IBD is a serious condition that often results in the need for major medical intervention:

> Crohn's disease alone accounts for 84,000 days of hospitalization and 1.3 million outpatient visits per year.

> About 70 percent of people with Crohn's need surgery to remove a diseased area of their intestines.

> About one-third of individuals with ulcerative colitis require surgery to have their colons removed.

> IBD costs the United States about $6.3 billion per year, and costs each patient an average of $8,000 per year.

the bowel is inflamed so as to balance motility, or the movement of food through the digestive tract. This means that the diarrhea that is a major symptom in IBD may become less frequent with CBD use.

Cannabis versus Other Treatments

The first line of defense for IBD treatment in mainstream medicine is anti-inflammatory medication, which can include corticosteroids. You may be able to skip the nasty side effects of steroids by using medical marijuana or a CBD supplement.

Natural Partners for Cannabis

Neither medical marijuana nor CBD works alone to treat IBD. Integration with other holistic modalities is crucial for IBD management:

> **KNOW YOUR FOOD TRIGGERS.** Varying ways to eat have been recommended to treat IBD, including lowering FODMAPs (fermentable oligosaccharides, disaccharides, monosaccharides, and polyols, a collection of carbohydrates that can be poorly absorbed by the body), the specific carbohydrate diet, and an anti-inflammatory diet. The goal of all these food plans is to balance the dysfunctional gastrointestinal system. It is important to identify your individualized food triggers to avoid symptom flare-ups. Alcohol is a gastrointestinal irritant, so it is not recommended with IBD. You can consult a nutritionist who has experience integrating nutrition with cannabis.

> **TRY A PROBIOTIC.** Some studies link the addition of beneficial bacteria to IBD relief. Check with a healthcare practitioner about the optimal probiotic strain for your condition.

> **LET IT OUT.** Researchers believe that stress plays a big part in IBD flare-ups. Certainly, living with IBD can take an emotional toll. Do what you need to do to relax, whether that means joining a support group, enjoying silent meditation, or stretching it out with some morning yoga.

> **PAY ATTENTION TO SLEEP HYGIENE.** Getting adequate sleep is vital to managing IBD. It appears that sleep disturbance and the interruption of circadian rhythms may aggravate the symptoms of IBD.

INSOMNIA

> Insomnia is a disorder that prevents you from getting enough sleep by keeping you awake or waking you following a short period of sleep.

> Roughly 30 percent of all American adults have experienced insomnia, and 10 percent of those have severe enough insomnia to disrupt daily activities.

> CBD may relieve conditions that contribute to insomnia while it also acts as a sleep aid.

We have all been there: you drag your tired body into bed, ready for a good night's sleep, only to stare at the ceiling for what feels like forever. Or you wake up hours before your alarm goes off and cannot get back to sleep. Maybe you stay in bed, stubbornly determined to fall asleep, or maybe you get up and clean the kitchen until you feel tired again. Maybe you are one of nearly 9 million Americans who use prescription sleep aids. Integrating CBD with other lifestyle practices may help you get the restful sleep that your body craves and needs.

Inside Insomnia

Insomnia makes it difficult to fall asleep, stay asleep, or wake up feeling rested. Although everyone is different, adults generally need about seven hours of sleep each night for optimal functioning the next day. Many adults experience acute insomnia, which can last a few days or weeks, and many suffer from chronic insomnia, which lasts a month or longer. Lifestyle tweaks can help people get sleep habits back on track for better rest.

CAUSES

Insomnia can be a side effect of medications or of other conditions, such as sleep apnea or chronic pain. In many instances, not falling or staying asleep is the result of one of these common factors:

> **STRESS.** When you have a lot on your plate, it can be difficult to turn your brain off at bedtime. That makes it challenging to get a good night's sleep. Combine that with grief or depression and you have a recipe for chronic insomnia.

> **FLUCTUATING SCHEDULE.** If your work schedule is ever-changing or you change time zones, you may be disrupting your circadian rhythm—the internal clock that guides your sleep–wake cycle.

> **BAD HABITS.** Sometimes you get in the way of your own circadian rhythm by taking late naps, using your bed for work, binge-watching shows, or scrolling through social media. Keeping a regular sleep schedule and turning off electronic devices several hours before bedtime can help.

> **LATE-NIGHT SNACKS.** Eating too close to bedtime means you have less time for digestion before lying down. Some people who eat late at night experience heartburn or other physical discomfort, which interferes with sleep.

> **CAFFEINE.** Consuming caffeine in beverages and foods too close to your bedtime—which is defined as within about five hours

A Real Problem

Without enough sleep at night, your whole day suffers—from your mood to your work to your relationships. Sleep deprivation can also be hazardous to your health and the safety of others.

> Drowsy driving accounts for 1,500 deaths and 40,000 more injuries in the United States each year.

> Sleep deprivation experienced by doctors plays a part in the 100,000 hospital deaths caused by medical error.

> Getting fewer than five hours of sleep a night can increase your risk of developing diabetes, hypertension, and coronary heart disease, all of which can have fatal consequences.

In fact, insufficient sleep is considered a public health epidemic.

but can vary widely among individuals—can have a detrimental impact on the quality of your sleep. Interestingly, there is a genetic component to caffeine metabolism. Some people can consume caffeine at late hours and have zero issues with sleep; for others, any amount of caffeine gets in the way of sleep.

SYMPTOMS

Obviously, sleeplessness is the main symptom associated with insomnia. That can mean a few different issues, such as:

> Difficulty falling asleep
> Difficulty staying asleep
> Waking too early in the morning
> Not feeling rested after sleeping
> Feeling sleepy during the day

Insomnia can also lead to:

> Irritability
> Depression or anxiety
> Difficulty concentrating or remembering
> Making mistakes
> Having accidents
> Feeling stressed about sleep

Who Is at Risk?

Individuals with fluctuating schedules or a stressful day can experience a few sleepless nights. Biological factors can also increase your risk of developing chronic insomnia:

> **AGE.** Changes in sleep patterns and health as we age make insomnia more likely in older adults.

> **GENDER.** Hormonal shifts can trigger insomnia, making women more likely to experience it. The discomfort of PMS or pregnancy can keep you awake, as can the night sweats and hot flashes of menopause.

> **MENTAL HEALTH.** Mental health conditions such as anxiety, depression, and PTSD can make your mind race at night and interrupt your sleep.

> **PHYSICAL HEALTH.** Sometimes sleep is the remedy needed for pain, such as a headache, and yet pain can keep you up at night. If that pain is related to a chronic health condition such as multiple sclerosis, the risk of insomnia increases.

The CBD Answer

For insomnia, many cannabis clinicians recommend cannabis with THC, even a small amount. For individuals who do not have access to medical marijuana in their states, a CBD supplement at higher doses may help to encourage regular and restful sleep. Cannabis may also help with chronic inflammation and pain, which can interfere with the quality of sleep.

HOW TO USE IT

For most individuals, CBD has a biphasic response. In terms of insomnia, that typically means that lower doses stimulate and higher doses sedate. You will need to find your specific CBD sweet spot for encouraging sleep. Caveat: If you are taking any medications, be sure to consult a qualified healthcare professional before incorporating CBD into your sleep hygiene routine.

WHY IT WORKS

The endocannabinoid system is intimately involved with sleep. The endocannabinoids that we make fluctuate with the circadian rhythm. Cannabis with THC or whole plant CBD may tackle insomnia by:

> **REDUCING PAIN.** If pain keeps you up at night, cannabis may reduce the inflammation that is causing the pain, taking the edge off to allow you to get some shut-eye.

> **RELIEVING ANXIETY.** When stress and worry keep you awake, CBD can reduce anxiety to help lull you into sleep.

Making Connections

Exploring conditions related to insomnia may be helpful. You can learn more in the Anxiety Disorders (page 73), Chronic Pain (page 113), Depression (page 122), Menopause (page 173), and Post-Traumatic Stress Disorder (page 199) chapters.

CBD VERSUS OTHER TREATMENTS

When you have spent one too many nights lying awake in bed, you may ask your doctor for a prescription sleep aid. Many have disturbing side effects and are not meant to be used long term. On the other hand, CBD may help you reset your sleep cycle and could relieve underlying issues such as anxiety and inflammation.

Natural Partners for CBD

Integrating CBD with sleep-promoting habits can ensure quality rest:

> **MAKE IT SACRED.** Turn your bedtime into a ritual of relaxation that gets your body used to nodding off at the same time every night. Like babies, adults need sleep routines, too!

> **HAVE A CUP OF TEA.** While caffeine is a late-night no-no, relaxing with a cup of caffeine-free herbal tea made with soothing ingredients such as chamomile can encourage shut-eye.

> **USE RELAXING ESSENTIAL OILS.** Lavender and pinene are two terpenes that encourage relaxation and sleep. Certain cultivars of cannabis feature these chemicals.

> **MEDITATE.** Adding a meditation practice to your daily routine at any time of the day can promote sleep.

> **SLEEP IN A DARK, COOL ROOM.** Sleep is more deep and restful when the sleep setting is darkened and the temperature is cooler.

> **KEEP THE ELECTRONICS OUT OF THE BEDROOM.** The television is no longer the only electronic device invading the bedroom. Watch out for cell phones, laptops, tablets, book

Insomnia versus Alcohol

Think sleep is overrated? Think again. Studies show that sleep deprivation and alcohol intoxication cause the same level of impairment. Going 17 to 19 hours without sleep is equivalent to a blood alcohol concentration of 0.05 percent. Most states set the legal limit at 0.08 percent. Mixing the two—sleep deprivation and alcohol—is even worse. Drinking one beer on four hours of sleep has the same impact as drinking six beers after a full night's sleep. Adequate sleep is essential for optimal brain function.

readers, and who knows what else may be on the electronic horizon—all of which interrupt the body's circadian rhythm.

> **CONSIDER TARGETED SUPPLEMENTS.** Several supplements can be helpful in sleep promotion. The mineral magnesium can help with falling asleep, and the amino acid glycine can help with staying asleep. Melatonin, which is a hormone produced by the body that aids with sleep–wake cycles, can be taken as an occasional supplement.

Top Insomnia Triggers as You Age

You are more likely to develop a sleep disorder as you get older, and there is good reason for that. Your circadian rhythm has to contend with changes in:

> **Sleep patterns.** Although you still may need seven hours of sleep, you might begin to naturally need to fall asleep earlier and wake earlier. Your sleep may also be a little restless, making you more likely to wake easily in the middle of the night.

> **Activities.** Most people are less active as they age, which can negatively impact sleep. And the less active you are, the more likely you are to take a sleep-disrupting nap.

> **Health.** Overall health can certainly affect how well you sleep. For example, some health conditions result in nocturia, or urinating at night. These conditions include urinary tract infections and prostate enlargement.

> **Medications.** Insomnia is a side effect of multiple medications that are commonly prescribed to individuals as they age.

IRRITABLE BOWEL SYNDROME

> Irritable bowel syndrome (IBS) is considered a functional disorder that results in disruptive digestive upset and discomfort.

> The condition affects up to 45 million people in the United States.

> Women are twice as likely as men to develop IBS and less likely to report symptoms to a doctor.

> CBD may be effective in reducing the symptoms associated with IBS.

Bloating, cramping, constipation, and ever-unpredictable diarrhea are hallmarks of IBS. The constant gastrointestinal discomfort experienced by individuals with IBS can interfere with everyday life. CBD may be able to offer relief and a better quality of living.

Inside IBS

IBS is a chronic condition that involves the large intestine. For most individuals, IBS can be managed with lifestyle habits.

CAUSES

The endocannabinoid system is intimately involved in gut health. Cannabis researcher and physician Ethan Russo believes that clinical endocannabinoid deficiency may contribute to IBS development.

Other factors that contribute to IBS include:

> **MUSCLE CONTRACTIONS.** Your intestines are lined with layers of muscle that contract as food passes through—a process referred to as gut motility. A balance between contractions in both strength and length is important for proper digestion. In people with IBS, that balance is dysregulated.

> **MISFIRING NERVES.** Crossed signals between the brain and digestive system may cause the nerves to overreact to normal changes, resulting in unnecessary pain and digestive dysfunction.

> **GUT-IMMUNE CONNECTION.** Studies have demonstrated an increased number of immune cells in the intestines of individuals with IBS.

> **BACTERIAL OVERGROWTH.** Research has shown that the microbiome in the small intestines of individuals with IBS is unbalanced, a condition referred to as dysbiosis.

> **INFECTION.** Some people develop IBS as the result of a bacterial or viral infection.

> **FOOD POISONING.** People who get food poisoning can have the same bacterial overgrowth that can occur in IBS. Plus, food poisoning can worsen symptoms of existing IBS.

> **LACTOSE AND GLUTEN INTOLERANCES.** People who have IBS have a greater chance of both lactose and gluten intolerance.

A Real Problem

Unpredictable IBS symptoms can interfere with work, relationships, and activities of daily living, with alarming statistics:

> A survey revealed that individuals with functional GI disorders would give up 25 percent of their lives (which averaged 15 years) and 14 percent would risk a one-in-1,000 chance of death to live without IBS symptoms.

> IBS affects between 25 and 45 million Americans or more, estimated at 10 percent of the world's population.

> Individuals who have IBS may spend years—6.6 on average—with symptoms before being diagnosed.

> **MENSTRUATION.** Women who have IBS experience more severe symptoms during their periods.

SYMPTOMS

IBS is a finicky condition whose symptoms are super-specific to the individual and can vary constantly. Some days the symptoms can be unbearable and other days completely absent. Common IBS symptoms include:

> Abdominal pain

> Cramping

> Bloating

> Excess gas

> Diarrhea

> Constipation

> Mucus in the stool

Sometimes IBS symptoms can be relieved with a bowel movement. Be sure to make an appointment with a healthcare professional if symptoms are severe to rule out more serious conditions, such as inflammatory bowel disease (see page 156) or even colon cancer.

Top IBS Triggers

Because the GI system in individuals is extra-sensitive to stimuli, it is important to avoid foods that trigger flare-ups, such as:

> Foods high in FODMAP (fermentable oligosaccharide, disaccharide, monosaccharide, and polyol) molecules, such as wheat and garlic

> Highly processed foods, such as cookies, chips, and sugary cereals

> Fried foods

> Carbonated drinks

> Coffee

> Alcohol

A good way to figure out what triggers your symptoms is to keep a journal of the foods you eat and your bowel movements, along with any symptoms, your mood, possible stress-inducing events, and any other possible factors. You can consult with a nutritionist who integrates CBD with food to help you develop your personal journal.

Who Is at Risk?

Anyone can develop IBS—men, women, children, old, and young. But a few factors can increase your risk:

> **AGE.** IBS is more likely to afflict people under 50.

> **GENDER.** Women are twice as likely to suffer from IBS—especially those undergoing estrogen replacement therapy, which suggests there may be a hormonal component.

> **FAMILY HISTORY.** IBS tends to run in families, so having a close relative with the condition puts you at higher risk of developing it.

The CBD Answer

Throughout history, cannabis has been used to treat gastrointestinal disorders. CBD can reduce the inflammation associated with IBS and alleviate the associated anxiety. A daily supplement integrated with good nutrition practices may help with IBS.

HOW TO USE IT

Along with an appropriate food plan and stress-reducing techniques, a daily dose of CBD taken as an oil or possibly in an edible is preferred for treating IBS. For more immediate relief during IBS flare-ups, using a vaporizer with CBD may be warranted. Consulting with a credentialed nutritionist who has experience integrating cannabis with food for IBS is recommended.

WHY IT WORKS

Ethan Russo's hypothesis is that we all have an underlying endo-cannabinoid tone, which is the combination of the status of your endocannabinoids and endocannabinoid receptors. (For a deeper discussion of this concept, see page 22.) To demonstrate the theory, consider that three health conditions that frequently occur

Making Connections

Exploring conditions related to IBS may be helpful. You can learn more in the Anxiety Disorders (page 73), Chronic Inflammation (page 108), and Inflammatory Bowel Disease (page 156) chapters.

together—IBS, fibromyalgia, and migraine—all appear to be impacted by the endocannabinoid system (ECS). The ECS affects multiple systems in the body, including the gastrointestinal, immune, and nervous, all of which play a role in IBS. CBD may help to balance clinical endocannabinoid deficiency and reduce symptoms of IBS.

CBD VERSUS OTHER TREATMENTS

So much of treating IBS is managing its symptoms, which makes CBD an excellent addition to an IBS treatment plan. By supporting your digestive, immune, and neurological health, CBD may increase the power of lifestyle choices to reduce flare-ups and relieving symptoms.

Natural Partners for CBD

IBS is a chronic condition, which means that management focuses on lifestyle choices. In addition to adding a CBD supplement, here are a few ways to reduce flare-ups:

> **CHANGE WHAT YOU EAT.** For some individuals, following a low-FODMAP food plan can reduce the symptoms of IBS.

The Truth about IBS

As a society, we have been conditioned to avoid conversation about bowel movements, which are literally the last part of the process in the movement of food through the digestive system. Avoiding this topic has contributed to myths surrounding IBS, but the truth is:

> **IBS is not overdiagnosed.** One pervasive myth is that doctors lump all patients with digestive issues into an IBS diagnosis. Although there are no tests—yet—to help diagnose the condition as a clinical endocannabinoid deficiency, an IBS diagnosis still adheres to a specific set of parameters.

> **IBS is not a psychological condition.** There is no doubt that stress can worsen IBS symptoms, as it does many symptoms. Sadly, many conventional practitioners treat IBS with anxiety and depression meds.

> **IBS is treatable.** Too many IBS patients have been told there is nothing they can do about the condition. Treating IBS, which is typically chronic, can mean avoiding certain foods and activities.

- ➤ **EMBRACE BACTERIA.** Studies show that adding a probiotic to your daily regimen can relieve IBS symptoms. Be sure to consult with a practitioner about what probiotic strains are optimal for you.

- ➤ **REACH FOR MINT.** IBS sufferers who struggle with abdominal pain can try enteric-coated peppermint oil capsules, which have been shown to act as an anti-spasmodic and relieve pain.

- ➤ **MAKE USE OF MASSAGE.** Massaging your abdomen can relax the muscles, which can affect the arteries and help food move through the intestines.

- ➤ **GET SOME FEEDBACK.** Biofeedback is a therapeutic technique that uses electrical sensors to help individuals learn how to relax the body and manage pain.

- ➤ **TRY GUIDED IMAGERY.** Using this mind–body technique to evoke images that promote relaxation may alleviate the pain associated with IBS.

- ➤ **TURN TO QIGONG.** This Eastern mind–body approach uses gentle, focused movement to restore energy flow throughout the body, which can help with the healing process.

*I use Nature's Way Primadophilus

Reuteri great probiotic for colon colony also Stonyfield yogurt w/ live cultures

MENOPAUSE

> Menopause signifies the end of a woman's fertility and, with the decrease in estrogen, can trigger a whole host of symptoms.

> Menopause can also lead to a loss of bone density and an increased risk of heart attack and stroke.

> CBD may relieve the symptoms of menopause and reduce the risk of complications.

Menstruation is part of a woman's life cycle, and so is menopause. Woman can experience challenges in both time periods of their reproductive lives. During their potential childbearing years, women may experience PMS or infertility, for example. During menopause, some women have hot flashes, night sweats, irritability, mood swings, and weight gain—to name a few symptoms. Making lifestyle changes, along with supplementing with CBD, may help with managing the effects of menopause.

Inside Menopause

Menopause is a transitional time that every woman experiences when the ovaries stop producing eggs. It marks the end of the menstrual cycle, with symptoms such as irregular periods, insomnia, and mood changes. What incites the symptoms of menopause is a drop in estrogen and progesterone in the body, which can increase the risk of conditions such as heart disease, stroke, and osteoporosis.

CAUSES

Menopause is a natural part of aging, but a few factors can contribute to early menopause:

➤ **HYSTERECTOMY.** When the ovaries stop producing eggs, menopause begins. Not all hysterectomies involve removing the ovaries, but those that do can bring menopause about immediately.

➤ **CHEMOTHERAPY AND RADIATION.** Cancer therapies can sometimes bring your menstrual cycle to a temporary halt, triggering menopause.

➤ **EPILEPSY AND OTHER MEDICAL CONDITIONS.** In some women with epilepsy, menopause occurs a decade earlier due to effects of seizures on brain regions that control hormone release.

➤ **PRIMARY OVARIAN INSUFFICIENCY.** Some women—about 1 percent—experience premature menopause, thought to be brought on by ovaries that do not produce sufficient reproductive hormones.

➤ **IN VITRO FERTILIZATION (IVF) TREATMENTS.** Because the age of menopause is directly related to the number of eggs in the ovaries, and because IVF treatments involve harvesting eggs from the ovaries, the question remains as to whether IVF can trigger earlier menopause.

A Real Problem

Changes in mood, problems sleeping, and osteoporosis are three possible symptoms of menopause that can have a major impact on your life.

➤ Anxiety and depression account for billions of dollars in lost productivity.

➤ Sleep disorders account for tens of thousands of accidents and injuries every year.

➤ More bone fractures occur in postmenopausal women because of the decrease in estrogen, which protects bones.

Studies have demonstrated that CBD is effective in balancing mood, regulating sleep, preserving bone density, and improving bone fracture healing.

SYMPTOMS

Menopause is an individual experience, with symptoms including:

- Hot flashes and night sweats
- Chills
- Mood changes
- Weight gain
- Thinning hair
- Dry skin
- Problems sleeping
- Vaginal dryness
- Lack of sex drive

Who Is at Risk?

Menopause is a life stage all women go through. Certain factors can increase the risk of complications:

- **SMOKING.** The average age of menopause is about one and a half years earlier for women who smoke than their nonsmoking counterparts. Additionally, smoking can increase the risk of osteoporosis and heart disease, which are already possible complications of menopause.
- **OBESITY.** Weight gain can be a side effect of menopause. Women who enter menopause overweight, even just somewhat, have an even greater risk of heart disease, plus an additional risk of obesity-related conditions such as diabetes.
- **FAMILY HISTORY.** Having a family history of heart disease and osteoporosis can put you at an even greater risk of these conditions during menopause.

Top Hot Flash Triggers

Hot flashes are the most common and complained-about symptom of menopause. During a hot flash, a woman experiences an intense feeling of warmth that can last anywhere from a few seconds to a few minutes; when they happen at night they are called night sweats. Hot flashes affect about 75 percent of menopausal women for about one or two years, but can continue for 10 years or longer. Various factors that can bring about hot flashes include:

- Stress
- Caffeine
- Alcohol
- Certain foods
- Heat
- Cigarette smoke

The CBD Answer

Roughly 60 percent of women experience mild menopausal symptoms, and 20 percent more have no symptoms at all. That makes CBD all the more effective as a wellness solution for women. The effects of lower estrogen during menopause, which can contribute to the development of heart disease and bone-density loss, may be reduced by the integration of CBD with other lifestyle habits.

HOW TO USE IT

The most commonly recommended way to use CBD as a wellness supplement is as an oil that you take sublingually, or under the tongue. Be sure to consult with a health professional about products, especially if you are taking medications.

WHY IT WORKS

As estrogen levels drop, the endocannabinoid system becomes less active, which can lead to changes in mood. Also, a decrease in endocannabinoid system signaling may be related to the hot flashes experienced during menopause. Cannabinoid receptors are involved with both menopause and osteoporosis. CBD may help menopausal women find relief from:

> **MOODINESS.** Researchers have found that CBD directly activates serotonin receptors and is potentially as effective as anti-anxiety medications in balancing mood.

> **SLEEPLESSNESS.** Taking CBD one hour before bedtime may relieve anxiety that is contributing to insomnia and thus promote longer and more restful sleep. For some people, cannabis with THC is more effective for sleep issues.

> **BONE-DENSITY LOSS.** Several promising studies show that CBD may help reverse the loss of bone density and protect the health of the skeletal system.

Making Connections

Exploring conditions related to menopause may be helpful. You can learn more in the Anxiety Disorders (page 73), Depression (page 122), Heart Disease (page 151), Insomnia (page 161), and Osteoporosis (page 194) chapters.

> **WEIGHT GAIN.** When combined with an optimal food plan and movement activities, CBD may help individuals achieve a healthy weight.

CBD VERSUS OTHER TREATMENTS

The most common treatment for menopause symptoms is hormone replacement therapy (HRT), which is intended only for short periods of time. Long-term HRT use can increase the risk of heart attack, blood clots, stroke, and certain cancers. Many doctors prescribe antidepressants, sleep aids, and other medications to menopausal women, all of which come with risky side effects. Adding CBD to lifestyle changes during menopause may reduce the need for pharmaceuticals.

Natural Partners for CBD

Menopause is both natural and temporary, so a holistic treatment plan can work well. In addition to adding a CBD supplement:

> **FOLLOW A WELLNESS ROUTINE.** Regular exercise and an optimal food plan can improve your mood, sleep, and health.

> **MAINTAIN GUT HEALTH.** Keeping your digestive system in order with an appropriate food plan and probiotics is a good practice. Consult with a professional to integrate nutrition with CBD.

> **GET SOME SUN.** Or, better yet, take a regular vitamin D supplement to ward off depression, maintain bone health, support weight management, and more.

> **TAKE A DEEP BREATH.** Practicing breathing through discomfort can help, especially with hot flashes.

> **MEDITATE.** A daily routine that features meditation can help you cope with the hills and valleys of menopause.

The Truth about Timing

Menopause is a transitional period, not a condition *per se*. You are considered menopausal when you have gone 12 months without a period; prior to that time you are in the perimenopausal phase. Some women experience symptoms of menopause for up to 10 years, others only a few months. On average, the transition lasts four years.

MIGRAINE

> ➤ Migraines can cause debilitating pain and be accompanied by nausea and sensitivity to everyday sights and sounds.

> ➤ More than 39 million people in the United States suffer from migraines, resorting to medications that are frequently ineffectual.

> ➤ Taking a daily CBD supplement may provide relief and reduce the frequency of migraines.

If you have ever had a migraine, you know that it is not just a headache. You cannot take a regular pain reliever and get back to work. With hallmarks including intense pain, light and sound intolerance, and nausea, migraines can be debilitating. And worse, a single migraine can last up to three days! Chronic migraine sufferers can spend more than half of every month in pain.

Prescribed treatments range from oral medications—meant to be both preventive and pain-relieving—to Botox injections (yes, you read that right!). Because migraines are somewhat of a medical mystery and these medications have serious side effects, scientists are still searching for better options. In the meantime, many sufferers have turned to "alternative" therapies such as food-sensitivity testing and supplements for relief. Cannabis is the newest—and a very promising—alternative.

Inside Migraines

Surprising but true: no one really knows what a migraine is, only what symptoms it can trigger. Scientists have theories, but they do not know *why* a person's pain receptors suddenly go on full alert. Researchers believe that migraines may be caused by two factors:

> **A KIND OF FAULTY WIRING** between the brainstem and the trigeminal nerve, which is the main nerve that carries pain impulses from the face and head to the central nervous system. This pathway disruption may cause individuals to become overly sensitive to pain stimuli, resulting in migraine.

> **A DROP IN THE LEVELS OF SEROTONIN,** which may cause the trigeminal nerve to release substances that bring about migraine pain.

The end result is intense, often unpredictable, pain.

CAUSES

Certain triggers—foods, hormones, events—can precede migraines. Common ones include red wine, sharp cheddar cheese, stressful situations, and loud environments. For some people, just sleeping in on the weekend can cause a migraine. Each individual has a different combination of triggers, some of which are unique to the person. Clinical endocannabinoid deficiency, described in more detail on pages 21–22, may contribute to the development of migraines. Clearly, the condition can seriously impact day-to-day life, aside from the actual migraine occurrences.

SYMPTOMS

Migraines can create a various symptoms, ranging from annoying to excruciating. The most common ones include:

> Intense, throbbing pain, frequently concentrated on one side of the head

> Sensitivity to light, sounds, and smells

> Nausea, and sometimes vomiting

> Visual disturbances

> Paresthesia, or a burning sensation in the extremities

Making Connections

Exploring conditions related to migraine may be helpful. You can learn more in the Chronic Pain (page 113) and Nausea (page 190) chapters.

Who Is at Risk?

Migraines are an equal-opportunity condition, affecting more than 39 million people in the United States alone. More than 4 million of those people suffer from chronic migraines, meaning they are in pain more than 15 days a month. In fact, the condition is so common that people who suffer from migraines have their own moniker: *migraineur*. A few factors affect those who may be more prone to attacks, including:

> **AGE.** Migraines tend to crop up during adolescence, get worse during your 30s, and gradually get better after age 50.

> **GENDER.** Migraines are significantly more prevalent in women than in men, with three times as many female sufferers. Women are especially likely to experience an attack when hormone levels drop just before their periods. Menopause and pregnancy can bring on an attack in women who have previously never had migraines.

> **GENETICS.** A family history of migraines increases the risk, and genetic anomalies have also been identified in individuals with chronic migraine.

Cannabis researcher and neurologist Ethan Russo has theorized that clinical endocannabinoid deficiency contributes to migraines. With more people diagnosed every day, the need for better treatment options grows.

The CBD Answer

Both cannabis with THC and whole plant CBD can be effective in dealing with chronic pain, so using cannabis for migraines makes sense. Many cannabis clinicians believe that migraine is best addressed by using cannabis with THC in small amounts.

The Truth about Migraine Meds

Many medications that are prescribed for migraines are "off-label" prescriptions, meaning originally intended to treat a different condition. For example, sometimes pharmaceuticals meant to treat seizures are prescribed for migraines because of observed benefits.

HOW TO USE IT

Because clinical endocannabinoid deficiency may be a contributing factor in migraine attacks, it may be wise for migraineurs to incorporate either cannabis with THC or whole plant CBD into their daily wellness routines. For possible immediate relief during an active attack, vaping is one of the most direct delivery methods.

WHY IT WORKS

Studies have found that migraine sufferers have lower levels of the endocannabinoid anandamide, the so-called bliss molecule. This

---

Common Migraine Triggers

> ➤ Foods, especially aged cheeses and highly processed foods, though food triggers are specific to the individual and may be evaluated with food-sensitivity testing

> ➤ Lack of food and skipping meals

> ➤ Food additives, such as the artificial sweetener aspartame and the flavor enhancer monosodium glutamate, or MSG

> ➤ Alcohol, particularly red wine

> ➤ Highly caffeinated beverages

> ➤ Withdrawal from caffeine

> ➤ Hormonal changes, particularly estrogen drops experienced by women during menstruation, pregnancy, breastfeeding, and menopause

> ➤ Stress, stress, stress

> ➤ Lack of sleep or too much sleep

> ➤ Jet lag

> ➤ Environmental factors, such as barometric pressure, mold, and pollen

> ➤ Excessive stimuli, such as loud noises, strong smells, and bright lights

> ➤ Medications, such as oral contraceptives and vasodilators

> ➤ Muscle tension

> ➤ Intense physical exertion

> ➤ Sinus infections

---

supports Dr. Russo's theory of clinical endocannabinoid deficiency, which he illustrates by examining the comorbid conditions migraine, fibromyalgia, and IBS. CBD may help to balance clinical endocannabinoid deficiency and reduce the occurrence and severity of migraines.

Antiemetics, which are typically used to treat motion sickness and are effective against nausea and vomiting, can sometimes break the migraine. The fact that THC also works as an antiemetic plus pain reliever supports the use of marijuana in the treatment of migraine.

CBD VERSUS OTHER TREATMENTS

The side effects of conventional migraine treatments are often not much better than the actual symptoms of migraines. Over-the-counter medications can damage the heart, liver, and stomach when taken on a regular basis. Opioids carry the risk of addiction, of course. Injections can cause allergic reactions. And prescription meds can produce side effects that range from drowsiness to stroke. In stark contrast, whole plant CBD may be a more sensible and effective option for migraine pain relief.

Natural Partners for CBD

Integrating CBD with lifestyle practices can provide the optimal treatment plan for dealing with migraines, such as:

> **KEEP A DETAILED JOURNAL.** Track your daily habits—eating, sleeping, other activities—to help you notice patterns and mitigate triggers. A journal can help you determine your success with CBD as well.

Prodrome, Aura, and Post-drome

Before an attack, sometimes two days earlier, a migraine sufferer may notice neck stiffness, mood changes, constipation, food cravings, and frequent yawning—referred to as *prodrome*. About 30 percent of suffers also experience an *aura*, or visual disturbance, such as light flashes or bright spots. Auras can also involve sensory sensations, movement, and speech. Following a migraine, referred to as *post-drome*, individuals can experience a "migraine hangover," feeling confused, moody, dizzy, and weak, with continued sensitivity to stimuli.

- ➤ **CONSIDER TARGETED SUPPLEMENTS.** The B vitamin riboflavin, magnesium, CoQ-10, and the herb butterbur have been demonstrated to reduce migraines for some individuals.

- ➤ **PLAN IN PROBIOTICS.** Maintaining gut health is an important component of health. Eating foods that contribute to a balanced microbiome, such as fermented vegetables, kefir, and kombucha, and taking a probiotic supplement may help. Consult a healthcare professional versed in the gut–brain axis and healing with food and cannabis for specific recommendations.

- ➤ **GO FOR FOOD-SENSITIVITY TESTING.** Some people have sensitivities to multiple foods that trigger migraine episodes. Testing for these sensitivities can help to pinpoint ingredients and chemicals that contribute to migraines.

- ➤ **INCORPORATE MEDITATION.** Practicing mindfulness meditation has been shown to reduce migraine attacks. Brain-wave and imaging studies actually demonstrate that meditation can change brain structure and activity.

- ➤ **TRY ACUPUNCTURE.** Studies have found that individuals who received acupuncture reported fewer days with migraines and a lessening of their intensity.

- ➤ **TURN TO MASSAGE.** Among the benefits of massage are stress reduction and pain and muscle tension relief. Some migraineurs find that regular massage reduces the number of migraine attacks.

The positive effects of various mind–body techniques support the theory of clinical endocannabinoid deficiency. Meditation, acupuncture, and massage can all increase your production of endocannabinoids, possibly reducing the occurrence of migraine episodes.

A Real Problem

Millions of people are searching for relief from migraines, and it is no wonder why:

- ➤ A single migraine attack can last up to three days.
- ➤ Chronic sufferers spend *more than half* of every month in pain.
- ➤ An overwhelming 91 percent of sufferers miss work or cannot function normally during an attack.

That is why discovering new treatments is so important.

MULTIPLE SCLEROSIS

> ➤ Multiple sclerosis, or MS, is a degenerative disease that affects the brain and nervous system.

> ➤ MS is the most common autoimmune inflammatory disorder; however, accurately identifying individuals with MS is difficult, with incidence estimated at about 400,000 in the United States.

> ➤ As a neuroprotective and anti-inflammatory compound, CBD may be able to mitigate the symptoms of multiple sclerosis.

Multiple sclerosis starts off subtly. Your vision gets blurry sometimes. Maybe you are more tired than usual or feel dizzy occasionally. You may notice numbness or tingling in your limbs. None of these things necessarily worry you right off the bat. You go to see an eye doctor, who tells you that you need an MRI.

After the test, a neurologist delivers devastating news: you have MS, and it is incurable. All you can do is manage the barrage of symptoms that you are going to experience for the rest of your life. Cannabis with THC and CBD are showing promising results in studies that have evaluated its effectiveness in both slowing the progression of the disease and relieving its symptoms.

Inside Multiple Sclerosis

Multiple sclerosis causes the body to attack and destroy the protective myelin sheath that covers nerve fibers, which disrupts communication between the brain and the body. Symptoms include pain, fatigue, muscle spasms, and more. The most common type of MS is relapsing-remitting, in which flare-ups are followed by periods of remission. Other types include secondary-progressive, primary-progressive, and progressive-relapsing, which all feature a steadier progression and worsening of symptoms. Treatment focuses on lifestyle changes that may mitigate symptoms.

CAUSES

Multiple sclerosis is considered an autoimmune disease, which means that the immune system assaults its own tissues. In this case, the protective part of the neuron, myelin, is attacked. Myelin's insulating function allows communication between the body and brain to occur quickly and efficiently. When myelin is damaged in individuals who have MS, the communication pathways become ineffective, resulting in a number of issues. Genetics, exposure to toxins such as heavy metals and chemicals, infections, and food intolerance are some of the main triggers for autoimmune diseases—including multiple sclerosis.

SYMPTOMS

Symptoms of MS vary by person, by disease type, and by progression. Common symptoms include:

- Depression
- Difficulty concentrating
- Dizziness
- Fatigue
- Lack of coordination
- Loss of bowel or bladder function
- Memory loss
- Muscle spasms
- Numbness or weakness in the limbs
- Partial or complete vision loss
- Slurred speech
- Tingling or pain in the body
- Tremors
- Unsteadiness in walking

Who Is at Risk?

Although the exact cause of MS is unknown, researchers have uncovered links to several factors that increase your risk of developing the disease.

- **AGE.** MS can strike at any age but most often occurs between the ages of 15 and 60. Symptoms typically appear between the ages of 30 and 35. Those who are diagnosed when they are older tend to have a more progressive form of the disease.

- **GENDER.** Women are two to three times more likely to develop MS than men.

- **FAMILY HISTORY.** If a close relative has MS, risk increases.

- **RACE.** White people of Northern European descent have a higher risk of developing MS than Hispanics, Asians, and people of African descent.

- **CLIMATE.** MS is more common in temperate climates than in warmer regions.

- **INFECTIONS AND ILLNESSES.** Having Epstein-Barr (the virus that causes mono), thyroid disease, type 1 diabetes, or inflammatory bowel disease puts you at a slightly higher risk for MS.

- **SMOKING.** Smokers are more likely than nonsmokers to develop MS.

Top Triggers for Flare-ups

Symptoms of MS can appear at any time, but there are a few common triggers that people with MS should avoid:

- **Stress.** Reducing stress, which can lead to confusion and fatigue, is one way to help keep symptoms at bay.

- **Lack of rest.** Individuals with MS do not have the same buildup of energy reserves as those without MS, which means they need more rest more often to face the day.

- **Heat.** Individuals with MS are especially sensitive to heat.

- **Infection.** Infections may trigger roughly one-third of MS flare-ups.

The Cannabis Answer

With its neuroprotective and anti-inflammatory benefits, cannabis with THC has been shown to reduce some symptoms associated with MS. Scientists are hoping for even more promising results using both cannabis with THC and whole plant CBD.

HOW TO USE IT

Taking a CBD supplement on a regular basis is a possible key to relieving the symptoms of MS. Surveys indicate that about half of individuals with MS use cannabis to lessen pain, spasticity, fatigue, and depression. Using products that offer more rapid relief of symptoms, such as vaporized cannabis and sublingual tinctures, is recommended. Because MS is related to chronic inflammation, avoid any inflammatory ingredients—such as sugar—in CBD edibles.

WHY IT WORKS

When it comes to MS, cannabis with THC and CBD works on cannabinoid receptors in three ways:

➤ **AS A PAIN RELIEVER.** THC has been known to both activate the feel-good chemicals in the body and dull the pain receptors, making it an effective pain reliever for MS flare-ups.

➤ **AS AN ANTI-INFLAMMATORY.** Inflammation is the immune-system response to a threat, which means it is inflammation that is doing the nerve damage in MS patients. By reducing

---

A Real Problem

Multiple sclerosis not only affects a large number of people throughout the world, but it also continues to worsen and impact the individual's life in new ways.

➤ Up to 70 percent of people with relapsing-remitting MS develop secondary-progressive MS, which causes a steady progression of symptoms, sometimes without any periods of remission.

➤ As MS progresses, it affects a person's mobility. One-third of individuals will need a wheelchair, while others may need a cane or crutches to walk—often because of fatigue, weakness, or balance issues.

that inflammation and bringing the immune system back into balance, CBD may reduce flare-ups and slow the progression of the disease.

> **AS A NEUROPROTECTIVE.** CBD not only protects the nervous system from damage (including the damage caused by the immune system attacking the myelin) but can also help the body generate new neurons.

CBD VERSUS OTHER TREATMENTS

Disease-modifying therapies are the most common treatments for MS, and using them can slow its progression. But their use needs to be strictly monitored to avoid complications and side effects, such as flu-like symptoms, liver damage, and even cancer. Many of these medications focus on reducing inflammation early on in the disease's progression, which makes anti-inflammatory CBD a smart addition to a treatment plan.

Natural Partners for CBD

Because MS is incurable and everyday things can prompt flare-ups, lifestyle habits are essential to reducing the symptoms of MS. Integrated with a CBD supplement, these lifestyle practices may reduce the symptoms and restore balance:

> **GET IN YOUR FRUITS AND VEGETABLES.** A food plan loaded with leafy greens, sulfur-rich foods such as cruciferous vegetables (broccoli, Brussels sprouts, cabbage, kale, etc.), and deeply pigmented foods such as blueberries, will provide important nutrients and offer neuroprotective and detoxifying benefits.

> **EAT HIGH-QUALITY PROTEIN.** When it comes to protein, stick to grass-fed and -finished meats and wild fish, which are full of brain-boosting omega-3 fatty acids.

> **FEED YOUR GUT.** Support your microbiome by eating a whole-food diet, as well as fermented foods such as kimchi, kefir, and kombucha.

> **UNCOVER FOOD SENSITIVITIES.** It is best to keep a journal to determine what foods and ingredients may aggravate symptoms. Some people have issues with dairy, eggs, and soy, for example, while others do not.

- **TAKE YOUR SUPPLEMENTS.** Nutritional deficiencies can accelerate neuronal degeneration, so it is important to consume adequate levels of zinc, magnesium, biotin, folate, vitamins K, D, and A, fish oil, alpha-lipoic acid, and acetyl carnitine.

- **MOVE YOUR MUSCLES.** Movement activities that are tailored to needs and abilities are essential for keeping mobility and coordination intact. Physical therapy, stretching, and qigong can be a tremendous help, especially in the later stages of the disease.

- **BE KIND TO YOURSELF.** MS takes a huge toll on your emotional and mental well-being, so finding ways to cope with the disease on those levels is important. Talk to a therapist, make time for get-togethers with friends, or join a yoga retreat.

- **GET PLENTY OF REST.** MS sufferers need to recharge their batteries more often and more fully to cope with the disease itself in addition to everyday activities. Adequate sleep is vital for individuals with MS.

- **PRACTICE MEDITATION AND GUIDED IMAGERY.** Mind–body techniques can help to alleviate stress and promote relaxation.

The Truth about Sativex

Sativex is a cannabis-based medication that has been shown to relieve MS symptoms, including neuropathic pain, spasticity, muscle spasms, and sleep disturbances. Because it has a CBD:THC ratio of 1:1, it has yet to be approved in the United States, although that may change. It is worth noting, however, that patients who use Sativex complain of side effects such as dizziness, sleepiness, and a feeling of intoxication. Nonintoxicating CBD may be able to produce similar relief without unwanted side effects.

NAUSEA

> ➤ Nausea is that uncomfortable feeling of unease that makes you feel like you might need to vomit but does not always predict vomiting.

> ➤ Everyone has experienced nausea throughout their lifetime, but it is a considerable problem for people whose required medications cause it regularly.

> ➤ CBD can act as an antiemetic for nausea caused by a variety of factors and conditions.

Nausea feels like both physical and emotional agony when you are in the throes of it. As your stomach churns, discomfort meets anxiety about whether or not you need to find a receptacle. Feeling like you need to vomit might be even worse than actually getting it over with, which could provide temporary relief. And for those whose medications come with a side effect of nausea—such as cancer patients going through chemo—that feeling is ever-present. Studies show, though, that CBD might be able to provide relief from queasiness.

Special Note for Pregnant Women

While CBD itself is safe for pregnant women because cannabinoids are naturally occurring compounds in the body, CBD products can contain ingredients that pregnant women may want to avoid. Without regulation to ensure product safety, it is important to work with a healthcare practitioner well educated in cannabis.

Inside Nausea

Nausea and vomiting are natural protective responses in which the body recognizes that something does not belong and tries to get rid of it. When the body is reacting to something bad, such as food poisoning or an underlying illness, this response is essential to your health. But sometimes nausea is just an unnecessary side effect of necessary treatments and medications.

CAUSES

Nausea is caused by the body's reacting to something it considers harmful and wanting to expel it. This mechanism can be triggered naturally (as in food poisoning or pregnancy) or artificially (as a side effect of medication).

SYMPTOMS

Nausea is a symptom of the body's desire to expel something it sees as harmful. It produces feelings of unease, an upset stomach, and a discomfort at the back of the throat.

Who Is at Risk?

Nausea is a universal experience that needs no underlying cause, but several medical conditions can trigger it:

- Anxiety
- Cancer
- Crohn's disease
- Chronic pain
- Depression
- Eating disorders
- Heart disease
- Irritable bowel syndrome
- Migraine
- Pregnancy

The Truth about Serious Nausea

Most of the time, nausea is just an annoyance. Maybe you ate too much, or drank too much, or have just started a new medication that needs time to settle into your system. But sometimes nausea can indicate a truly serious condition, such as a heart attack or appendicitis. If you are not sure why you are feeling nauseated and you suspect something is really wrong, seek medical help immediately.

The CBD Answer

Whether you have a sensitive stomach or are working through chemo, CBD has the potential to soothe your stomach and help you feel normal again. Studies show that it is a powerful antiemetic, thanks to the endocannabinoid system's role in regulating both nausea and vomiting. Cannabis has been used to treat nausea in patients for a number of years and its efficacy is widely recognized.

HOW TO USE IT

If you suffer from frequent nausea, maybe because of a medication, you will want a low daily dose of CBD or stomach-soothing CBD-infused peppermint tea. If you need to, you can always work your way up to higher doses. For acute nausea (the kind that just suddenly shows up), try vaping CBD for quick relief. Since this method bypasses the GI tract, it is a good option for nausea sufferers.

WHY IT WORKS

The endocannabinoid system is far reaching in what it regulates, and researchers have linked it to the mechanisms of nausea and vomiting. CBD acts on cannabinoid receptors to both prevent and relieve nausea. CBD can increase levels of anandamide, an endocannabinoid, which supports homeostasis.

CBD VERSUS OTHER TREATMENTS

Medications used for nausea usually treat a specific root cause, such as motion sickness. But the medication that helps with motion sickness

Top Nausea Triggers

If you have ruled out a serious underlying illness, one of the following everyday factors might be bringing on your nausea:

- Alcohol consumption
- Food poisoning
- Medications (such as antibiotics)
- Migraine
- Motion sickness
- Overeating
- Pain (such as from a minor injury)
- Pregnancy
- Stress

will not help with other causes of nausea. CBD, however, acts on the nausea itself, not on any underlying cause. You can use it to gently treat any sort of condition causing nausea.

Natural Partners for CBD

In addition to taking a CBD supplement, you can find natural relief for nausea in a number of ways.

> **SOOTHE WITH A SPICE.** Ginger has been used to treat digestive issues for 2,000 years. Try consuming it as a tea to quickly relieve nausea.

> **TURN TO AGE-OLD PRACTICES.** Acupuncture and acupressure are staples of Eastern medicine that focus on stimulating pressure points throughout the body (with thin, painless needles or pressure) to release hormones that reduce feelings of pain and nausea.

> **TAKE A DEEP BREATH.** Breathing exercises and meditation can help you move your focus away from the nausea, effectively dulling it so that you do not notice the feeling.

A Real Problem

Although nausea is often nothing more than a temporary annoyance, it can be a long-term battle for people who suffer from it as a side effect.

> Nausea is one of the most common medication side effects reported.

> It can take both an emotional and a physical toll, lowering quality of life.

> Long-term nausea can result in loss of appetite, which leads to dehydration, malnutrition, and health complications. This makes it especially difficult to fight the condition for which you are taking medication.

OSTEOPOROSIS

> ➤ Osteoporosis is a common, usually age-related, condition that causes bones to weaken and become brittle.

> ➤ About 54 million Americans have or are at risk for osteoporosis, which can lead to pain and easily broken bones.

> ➤ Studies show that CBD can reduce bone loss and actually strengthen bones.

We take our bone health for granted, right up until a break. When you have osteoporosis, a break is much more likely, costly, painful, and serious. In severe cases, something as simple as sneezing can bring about a fracture. That is why it is so important to eat well, exercise, and take supplements—such as vitamin D, calcium, and CBD—that support bone health.

Inside Osteoporosis

We think of bone as rigid and static, but it is actually living tissue that is constantly aging, breaking down, and reforming. Osteoporosis occurs when new bone growth cannot keep up with bone loss, resulting in weaker structure overall. This can lead to fractures, especially in the hip, wrist, or spine.

CAUSES

We actually accumulate our greatest bone mass before we hit our early 20s. After that, bone loss naturally begins to outpace bone growth.

Having accumulated less bone at an early age can lead to osteoporosis later. So can a lack of exercise or proper nutrition, some medications, and hormone fluctuations.

TOP TRIGGERS OF BONE LOSS

An alarming number of conditions can increase your risk for bone loss, including:

> - Autoimmune disorders (rheumatoid arthritis, multiple sclerosis)
> - Digestive disorders (celiac disease, inflammatory bowel disease)
> - Cancer (specifically breast and prostate)
> - Blood disorders (leukemia and lymphoma)
> - Neurological disorders (stroke, Parkinson's disease)
> - Hormonal disorders (diabetes, hyperthyroidism)
> - Mental illness (depression, eating disorders)

SYMPTOMS

Osteoporosis can sneak up on you because you do not feel yourself losing bone. What you may notice instead is:

> - Back pain (caused by a fracture)
> - Loss of height
> - Curve in the back or stooped posture
> - An unexpected and seemingly unwarranted bone fracture

The Truth about Osteoporosis Meds

If you have been diagnosed with osteoporosis in the last 15 years or so, your doctor has probably prescribed you a bisphosphonate, which is a class of drug meant to preserve and build bone. But the long-term risks of these medications are starting to become clear—and starting to outweigh the benefits. It turns out that the drugs only ever helped a little bit more than placebos. Compare that with the side effects—serious gastrointestinal troubles, abnormal heart rhythm, and even a particular kind of fracture—and these meds may not be worth the trouble. Consider with your doctor if you can instead focus on holistic help, such as preventing falls and strengthening bones with diet and exercise.

Who Is at Risk?

A number of factors can increase osteoporosis risk, including:

- **AGE.** The older you get, the more bone loss outpaces bone growth and the higher your risk for osteoporosis.

- **GENDER.** Women are much more likely than men to develop the condition.

- **RACE.** People who are white or Asian have the highest risk of osteoporosis.

- **FAMILY HISTORY.** Having a close relative with osteoporosis—especially with a hip fracture—increases your risk.

- **SIZE.** Being small in stature can increase your risk because you had less bone growth to begin with.

- **POOR NUTRITION.** You need to feed your bones to help them regenerate, so a lack of proper nutrition and vitamins can increase your risk of osteoporosis.

- **LACK OF EXERCISE.** Bones need to be strengthened, especially as we get older. Being less active—as a child or as an adult—can put your bone density at risk.

- **CERTAIN MEDICATIONS.** A long list of medications, including corticosteroids, can cost you bone density. Check with your prescribing healthcare practitioner to see if you are at risk.

- **OTHER MEDICAL CONDITIONS.** See "Top Triggers of Bone Loss" for conditions that can put you at risk for osteoporosis.

A Real Problem

Osteoporosis is a serious condition, made worse by the fact that you cannot feel your bones getting weaker. Not only can it cause painful breaks, but it can actually lead to fatalities.

- Osteoporosis costs patients, their families, and the healthcare system $19 billion per year.

- One in two women and one in four men over the age of 50 will break a bone due to osteoporosis.

- Twenty-four percent of people over 50 who break a hip die from complications within a year.

The CBD Answer

More and more, studies are showing that CBD may hold hope for those with osteoporosis. Further research is needed, but researchers have found that CBD has the potential not only to stop bone loss but to stimulate the formation of new bone.

HOW TO USE IT

Taking a CBD supplement regularly is the key to supporting your bone health. You can use any delivery method that suits you, but start with a low dose and spread it out over each day. For the purposes of dosing, you will not know how much CBD is helping to strengthen your bones. Instead, watch for it to help with your overall well-being, increasing the dose in small increments until you find one that seems to make a difference for you.

WHY IT WORKS

The skeletal system is full of CB2 receptors, which CBD works on to protect against bone loss and even stimulate bone formation. Its antioxidant and anti-inflammatory properties also support a healthy immune system, which reduces the risk of conditions that can result in osteoporosis.

CBD VERSUS OTHER TREATMENTS

Medications that are meant to mitigate bone loss or strengthen bones can cause unwanted side effects, such as stomach upset. CBD can help strengthen bones without any harmful side effects, plus it can relieve the side effects of other medications.

Natural Partners for CBD

Improving your health naturally can go a long way toward combatting osteoporosis. In addition to taking a CBD supplement:

> **EAT WELL.** A diet rich in vitamins and minerals is extremely important for bone health. Be sure to incorporate foods high in calcium, vitamin D, vitamin K, magnesium, and omega-3 fatty acids into your food plan.

> **EXERCISE.** Focus on weight-bearing and muscle-strengthening exercises to help slow bone loss and prevent fractures.

➤ **TAKE YOUR VITAMINS.** Vitamin D and calcium are a package deal for bone health, and an important one at that. Your bones need calcium to grow, and your body needs vitamin D to help your bones absorb the calcium.

➤ **GET CHECKED REGULARLY.** Because osteoporosis sneaks up on you silently, it is important to get tested for it regularly if you have any of the risk factors associated with the condition. Health insurance will generally cover a test every two years.

POST-TRAUMATIC STRESS DISORDER

> ➤ Post-traumatic stress disorder, or PTSD, is a mental health disorder that occurs in individuals who experience or witness a traumatic event.

> ➤ Childhood trauma can be a series of events that may not seem traumatic from an adult's point of view, and may even have been forgotten, but still are affecting the psyche of the individual.

> ➤ At least 24.4 million Americans have been diagnosed with PTSD, and that number grows daily.

> ➤ CBD may reduce the anxiety and depression associated with PTSD while protecting the brain from damage.

Trauma is all too common in this world of ours. Between military action, killing sprees, terrorist attacks, accidents, natural disasters, and abusive relationships, traumatic events can impact us daily. Every person deals with trauma differently; although humans are overwhelmingly resilient, sometimes trauma can overwhelm. When that happens, post-traumatic stress disorder can appear with its panic attacks, nightmares, mood swings, depression, and more symptoms that get in the way of enjoying an active life. While the condition is complex and difficult to treat, cannabis and cannabinoids may be a powerful part of a PTSD treatment plan.

Inside PTSD

Post-traumatic stress disorder is characterized by uncontrollable anxiety and memory flashbacks to the traumatic event or events. It is most common in war veterans but can be the result of any kind of traumatic event. PTSD can affect and disrupt work, relationships, and everyday life, so it is important to find treatments that work.

CAUSES

PTSD is caused by witnessing or directly experiencing a traumatic event involving actual or threatened death, serious injury, or sexual violence. Two people with the same experience can have different reactions— one may develop PTSD and the other may not. A combination of factors may contribute to development of the disorder:

➤ The number of traumatic events experienced in a lifetime

➤ Inherited mental health risks

➤ Individual temperament

➤ Biological response to stress

SYMPTOMS

PTSD varies from person to person in both when and how symptoms show up. Symptoms may appear immediately following a traumatic event or may take years to appear. PTSD symptoms are usually severe enough to interfere with daily life. They are grouped into four categories:

➤ **INTRUSIVE MEMORIES.** These include flashbacks and nightmares.

A Real Problem

As we are exposed to longer-lasting wars and increased violence, PTSD is becoming more common. As of now:

➤ Roughly 223 million people have experienced a traumatic event in their lifetime.

➤ About 20 percent of victims of a severe traumatic event will develop PTSD.

➤ PTSD costs the United States $42.3 billion per year in healthcare costs plus workplace and mortality costs.

> **AVOIDANCE.** Sufferers may avoid thinking or talking about the traumatic event, as well as physically avoiding places and things that remind them of the event.

> **NEGATIVE CHANGES IN THINKING AND MOOD.** This set of symptoms includes hopelessness, detachment, memory problems, and difficulty maintaining relationships.

> **CHANGES IN PHYSICAL AND EMOTIONAL REACTIONS.** Being wary or easily startled, having trouble sleeping or concentrating, irritability, aggression, and guilt fall into this category.

Who Is at Risk?

Anyone can develop PTSD, but factors that can increase your risk include:

> **FAMILY HISTORY.** Having a close relative with mental health issues can increase the risk of developing mental health issues, including PTSD.

> **GENETICS.** Various genetic markers may increase risk.

> **WORK.** Having a job that increases your exposure to trauma is certainly a factor.

> **MENTAL HEALTH.** Experiencing anxiety or depression can trigger PTSD.

> **SUPPORT.** Lack of a support system for coping with trauma increases vulnerability.

> **LENGTH OF TRAUMA.** PTSD is more common in people who have experienced intense or long-lasting trauma.

Types of Traumatic Events

Though each person has a different emotional threshold for trauma, common traumatic events include:

> Exposure to combat
> Physical abuse during childhood
> Sexual violence
> Physical assault

> Being threatened with a weapon
> Being in a severe accident
> Experiencing a life-threatening event

> **OTHER TRAUMAS.** Experiencing other, similar traumas earlier in life can intensify a person's reaction to new trauma and increase the risk of PTSD.

The Cannabis Answer

Although PTSD can be challenging to treat and typically requires a combination of therapies, integrating cannabis with other lifestyle habits may help people to overcome the disorder. Cannabis may restore balance and homeostasis while acting as a neuroprotectant, anti-inflammatory, and anxiolytic without the side effects of conventional medications.

HOW TO USE IT

Work with a cannabis clinician who treats PTSD, especially if you are taking other medications, because of possible interactions. With PTSD it is important to keep blood levels of cannabinoids constant, so taking whole plant CBD or cannabis with THC consistently is important. Divide doses over the course of the day to help keep blood levels constant and for maximum effectiveness. You can also use a faster-acting delivery method such as vaping when needed. Again, working with a practitioner to find your sweet spot is recommended.

Too Much of Good Thing?

Some people with PTSD *overconsume* cannabis with THC. *Overdosing* on cannabis is not possible because we have very few endocannabinoid receptors in our brain stem, which is the area of our brain responsible for the autonomic functions of heart rate and breathing. However, overconsumption is possible and can result in endocannabinoid receptors becoming desensitized to the point that cannabis no longer works and larger doses are required. Read Less Is More on page 40 for more information.

Sometimes taking too much cannabis with THC can increase anxiety, so proceed with caution. Additionally, cannabis does not work for everyone with PTSD. Some people have a genetic predisposition whereby cannabis triggers anxiety, regardless of the amount. Testing for this genetic mutation is available from some specialty labs.

WHY IT WORKS

CBD can reduce the symptoms of PTSD by acting on the serotonin pathway. With nearly half of all individuals with PTSD already using cannabis, a large amount of anecdotal evidence points to its efficacy in treating overall symptoms, such as reducing flashbacks, increasing quality of sleep, and decreasing anxious feelings or thoughts. The endocannabinoid system has been shown to be involved with emotional memory and regulation of the stress response. Some research indicates that the endocannabinoid system can aid in the extinction of negative memories.

CBD VERSUS OTHER TREATMENTS

The most common conventional treatment for PTSD is a combination of psychotherapy and antidepressant or anti-anxiety medication. While psychotherapy can be extremely beneficial, the medications can have serious side effects. These can range from mild ones such as headache and nausea to more serious effects such as depression and dependency on the drug, so it is important to work with a healthcare practitioner to find the best treatment for you. CBD is believed to work like frequently prescribed anxiety medications but without the side effects, so it is a great option to explore.

The Truth about Combat-Related PTSD

Our military personnel are at high risk for developing PTSD, especially if they have witnessed active combat.

> ➤ Up to 30 percent of veterans have been diagnosed with PTSD.

> ➤ The number of diagnosed cases of PTSD in the military has recently increased by 50 percent.

> ➤ Studies estimate that one in five veterans returning from Iraq and/or Afghanistan has PTSD.

> ➤ Seventy-one percent of all female military personnel develop PTSD as a result of sexual assault or unwanted advances while serving.

PTSD is a serious, life-altering condition that requires support and understanding from healthcare professionals, friends, family, policy makers, health insurance companies, and humanity at large.

Natural Partners for CBD

PTSD can be challenging to overcome. Here are some ways to integrate CBD with other lifestyle habits to mitigate the symptoms:

> ➤ **CONSULT A MENTAL HEALTH COUNSELOR.** Make an appointment with a professional who can counsel you about coping with symptoms.

> ➤ **SHARE YOUR EXPERIENCE.** Talking to someone—a friend, family member, spiritual leader—about your experience can be helpful and validating.

> ➤ **CLEAN UP YOUR HABITS.** Self-medicating with substances, such as cigarettes, alcohol, opioids, sugar, and caffeine, is a real issue with PTSD. Getting clean from the inside out can help you take control of your mental health.

> ➤ **EAT FOR BRAIN HEALTH.** What happens in your gut, happens in your brain. Create a food plan that is loaded with vegetables of all colors, deeply pigmented berries, detoxifying herbs, restorative fats, and high-quality protein, and devoid of inflammatory ingredients such as sugar, artificial ingredients, and gluten. Seek the guidance of a nutrition professional well versed in diets for promoting the gut–brain axis.

> ➤ **FIND OUTLETS.** Breaking the cycle of anxiety is important in overcoming PTSD, and having something that makes you happy and distracts you can help. Find an activity or hobby that is meaningful to you. Some ideas include pottery, mountain climbing, volunteering, coaching a children's team, joining a band, and knitting.

> ➤ **TRY YOGA.** Yoga and meditative practices can help you channel potential fear and stress stimuli in a safe space. Physiological triggers for a PTSD episode often involve heavy breathing or an increase in heart rate, so training your body to be mindful of such triggers may help.

PREMENSTRUAL SYNDROME

> Premenstrual syndrome (PMS) is a cluster of symptoms that most women experience in response to a drop in estrogen and progesterone levels after ovulation.

> More than 90 percent of women report PMS symptoms, which can include back pain, bloating, headaches, fatigue, and irritability.

> CBD may offer mood-balancing, anti-inflammatory, and pain-relieving effects to reduce a number of PMS-related symptoms.

Several days or maybe a week before your period starts, everyday irritations may be magnified and you might become bloated and more emotional. For women who experience PMS, integrating CBD into their wellness routine may be an excellent option to alleviate symptoms.

Inside PMS

Premenstrual syndrome is actually a collection of symptoms related to a time period before menstruation starts each month. After ovulation, estrogen and progesterone levels drop dramatically, causing a range of physical and emotional effects such as fatigue, mood swings, head-aches, and digestive issues.

CAUSES

In addition to the drop in hormones experienced before menstruation, a few other theories have been offered:

> **CHEMICAL CHANGES IN THE BRAIN.** Fluctuations in serotonin, the feel-good chemical, may trigger PMS symptoms such as fatigue, food cravings, and depression.

> **UNDIAGNOSED DEPRESSION.** Women with undiagnosed depression may notice an increase in intensity around their periods and attribute that to PMS alone.

> **THE ENDOCANNABINOID ANANDAMIDE.** The uterus boasts the highest concentration in the body of the endocannabinoid anandamide, linking the endocannabinoid system and the female reproductive system. Estrogen boosts production of anandamide—the "bliss molecule"—as well as cannabinoid receptors. When estrogen levels are at their lowest just prior to menstruation, anandamide levels are also at their lowest.

SYMPTOMS

PMS symptoms typically appear about five days before menstruation and dissipate as hormone levels rise with the beginning of menstruation. They can include:

> Acne

> Alcohol intolerance

> Anxiety

> Bloating

> Brain fog

> Breast tenderness

> Constipation or diarrhea

> Depression

> Food cravings

> Emotional lability, particularly crying

> Fatigue

> Headache

> Insomnia

> Irritability

> Low libido

> Muscle pain

> Weight gain

Making Connections

Exploring conditions related to PMS may be helpful. You can learn more in the Anxiety Disorders (page 73), Depression (page 122), and Insomnia (page 161) chapters.

Who Is at Risk?

Any woman who menstruates is at risk for premenstrual syndrome, and there are several other risk factors:

> **AGE.** The life stage between menarche, when a young woman begins to menstruate, and menopause, when ovulation ends, is when PMS can occur.

> **STRESS.** Women who report higher levels of daily stress and anxiety experience PMS more frequently.

> **ANXIETY AND DEPRESSION.** Women with anxiety disorders or depression have a greater incidence of PMS.

> **TRAUMA.** Experiencing trauma increases the chances of experiencing PMS and a more severe version, premenstrual dysphoric disorder (PMDD).

> **ALCOHOL INTAKE.** Studies have shown that women with PMS drink significantly more alcohol.

> **SMOKING.** Smokers appear to experience PMS more than their nonsmoking counterparts.

> **OBESITY.** Population-based studies have revealed a correlation between a body mass index of over 30 with PMS.

The CBD Answer

Because CBD interacts indirectly with the whole endocannabinoid system to restore balance, it can relieve many of the symptoms of PMS, including discomfort, anxiety, acne, digestive issues, and insomnia.

The Male PMS

Yes, there appears to be a version of PMS for males, referred to as irritable male syndrome, or IMS. The symptoms include general moodiness, anxiety, depression, and low self-esteem. Whereas PMS is triggered by a drop in estrogen and progesterone, IMS is triggered by a drop in testosterone. IMS, however, does not occur at a prescribed time of the month—it can occur at any time. That is because testosterone levels can fluctuate throughout the day, every day. So the next time the men in your life start getting on your case for PMS, remind them that they have their mood swings, too.

HOW TO USE IT

A low daily dose of CBD is usually enough to take the edge off of PMS. You can take this in smaller doses throughout the day to extend relief and use whatever delivery method you like. Some CBD-infused dark chocolate may just kill two birds with one stone—helping to regulate symptoms while satisfying cravings. For best results, take the supplement every day throughout the month, not just on days you experience symptoms.

WHY IT WORKS

The endocannabinoid system, or ECS, and the female reproductive system, which involves hormone fluctuations, are intertwined. CBD may help to balance the ECS and help with multiple symptoms:

> **ANXIETY AND DEPRESSION.** Research shows CBD directly activates serotonin receptors.

> **DIGESTIVE ISSUES.** The diarrhea and constipation that can occur may be triggered by fluctuating hormone levels, by anxiety, or by inflammation—all of which CBD may help.

> **PAIN AND DISCOMFORT.** CBD may be even more powerful than popular anti-inflammatories such as ibuprofen.

CBD VERSUS OTHER TREATMENTS

Over-the-counter pain relievers and mood-enhancing meds, which are frequently prescribed to women with PMS, often come with serious side effects, including liver damage. Integrated with optimal lifestyle habits, CBD may be able to provide symptom relief that is more effective and free of serious side effects.

Natural Partners for CBD

Relieving the symptoms of PMS can make an enormous difference in a woman's life. Combining a CBD supplement with other lifestyle habits can help to optimize PMS symptom relief:

> **CONSIDER TARGETED SUPPLEMENTS.** Nutritional supplements including evening primrose oil, vitamin B_6, magnesium, and certain herbs may alleviate PMS. Be sure to consult with a women's health practitioner who is competent in both nutrition and CBD for recommendations.

- **MOVE YOUR BODY.** Getting adequate movement may mitigate PMS symptoms, such as depression, fatigue, and brain fog.

- **EAT A WHOLE-FOOD DIET.** PMS cravings may lead you to consume highly processed foods. Following a diet of whole, unprocessed or minimally processed foods may help to keep symptoms at bay.

A Real Problem

Unfortunately, PMS is frequently minimized or dismissed in patriarchal society. Movies depict male characters asking women who assert themselves if it is "that time of the month." PMS is no laughing matter. It comes with real and sometimes serious physical and emotional symptoms that affect the majority of women. In fact: Over 90 percent of women experience premenstrual syndrome. There are about 200 different symptoms of PMS, and each woman experiences her own unique combination.

Women who suffer from depression, as well as those who have suicidal tendencies, may experience more severe symptoms as a result of mood fluctuation triggered by PMS.

PSORIASIS

> ➤ Psoriasis is a common skin condition that causes the buildup of extra skin cells that form itchy and uncomfortable scales or red patches on the surface of the skin.

> ➤ About 7.5 million Americans suffer from psoriasis, making it the most common autoimmune disease in the United States.

> ➤ CBD's anti-inflammatory effects can slow the overgrowth of skin cells that causes this skin condition.

A woman reaches for the top shelf at the supermarket and you see scaly red patches on her arm. How do you react? If you've seen one of the half-dozen pharmaceutical ads for psoriasis treatments, you may understand that what you see isn't a contagious illness but a painful skin condition.

A Real Problem

Psoriasis is much more than a "cosmetic" problem. In fact:

> ➤ Nearly 60 percent of individuals with psoriasis report that it interferes with their quality of life.

> ➤ As many as 30 percent of people with psoriasis develop psoriatic arthritis, a condition that causes painful, swollen joints.

> ➤ People with psoriasis are 15 to 20 percent more likely to suffer from depression because of the strain of living with the condition.

Types of Psoriasis

The type of psoriasis varies by how and where it strikes. Types include:

➤ **Plaque.** This is the most common kind of psoriasis, with dry, raised, red plaques that show up anywhere on the body—including inside the mouth.

➤ **Nail.** Psoriasis that affects the fingernails and toenails can cause abnormal growth and discoloration.

➤ **Guttate.** Usually caused by a bacterial infection such as strep throat, guttate psoriasis creates small lesions on the body, arms, legs, and scalp of children and young adults.

➤ **Inverse.** This type of psoriasis causes smooth patches of inflamed skin in the armpits, around the groin, and under the breasts.

➤ **Pustular.** This uncommon type of psoriasis causes large patches of pus-filled blisters.

➤ **Erythrodermic.** The worst and, thankfully, least common type, erythrodermic psoriasis covers the entire body with a painful rash.

➤ **Psoriatic arthritis.** In addition to having plaques on the skin, people with psoriatic arthritis suffer from painful, inflamed joints, though not necessarily at the same time.

Inside Psoriasis

Psoriasis is a chronic condition that speeds up the life cycle of skin cells. As cells proliferate, they form itchy, painful scales and inflamed patches on the skin's surface. Treatments focus on slowing down cell growth and managing the symptoms of flare-ups with lifestyle changes.

CAUSES

Psoriasis is an autoimmune disease, which means that it results from a person's own immune system attacking their body. Scientists aren't sure why it happens, but they have a theory: overactive T cells.

T cells are meant to travel through the body, defending it from infections. But in psoriasis, T cells attack healthy skin and "heal" the perceived wound by increasing the production of new skin cells. The skin cells move to the surface too quickly, forcing the T cells to start all over and continue the cycle until treatments put a stop to the skin lesions, or plaques, or they stop on their own.

SYMPTOMS

Psoriasis symptoms come and go as the condition flares up and then goes into temporary remission. Depending on the type of psoriasis and the individual, symptoms can include:

- ➤ Red patches of skin covered with silvery scales
- ➤ Small scaly spots, common in children
- ➤ Dry, cracked, sometimes bleeding skin
- ➤ Scaly skin, itching, and pain around the eyes
- ➤ Itching
- ➤ Burning
- ➤ Soreness
- ➤ Thick, pitted, or ridged nails
- ➤ Joint pain

Who Is at Risk?

Researchers don't know what triggers overactive T cells, but they believe it may have to do with one or more of the following factors:

- ➤ **FAMILY HISTORY.** Having close relatives—especially parents—with psoriasis can increase your odds of developing the disease because there is a genetic link.
- ➤ **INFECTIONS.** People with HIV or a recurring infection such as strep throat are more likely to develop psoriasis.
- ➤ **STRESS.** Having higher-than-normal stress levels can affect your immune system, which can increase your risk of developing psoriasis.

Making Connections

Exploring conditions associated with psoriasis may be helpful. You can learn more in the Anxiety Disorders (page 73) and Depression (page 122) chapters.

- **OBESITY.** Excess weight can increase your risk because skin folds provide a home for plaques.

- **SMOKING.** Smoking may cause you to develop psoriasis and usually increases the severity of the disease.

The CBD Answer

A hallmark of CBD is its ability to activate receptors in the immune system to restore balance and normal functionality. Research has shown that cannabinoids can inhibit skin-cell proliferation, which contributes to the flaky, red skin seen in individuals with psoriasis. CBD may quell the inflammation associated with psoriasis and help with the anxiety and depression associated with the condition.

HOW TO USE IT

You can use CBD to treat psoriasis in two ways:

- **AS A SUPPLEMENT.** To reduce the number of flare-ups, stretch the dose out over the course of the day for maximum effectiveness.

- **AS A TOPICAL TREATMENT.** Apply a CBD-infused cream to red, itchy skin whenever needed. Look for products that also feature other appropriate ingredients, such as aloe vera and moisturizers.

WHY IT WORKS

CBD helps psoriasis sufferers by acting on cannabinoid receptors in the skin to:

- Reduce inflammation at the source
- Reduce the overproduction of skin cells
- Dull the body's response to the pain caused by psoriasis flare-ups
- Increase the release of serotonin and boost overall happiness

CBD VERSUS OTHER TREATMENTS

The first line of defense in treating psoriasis is usually topical creams, which can relieve itching and irritation but are only meant for flare-ups. Taking a CBD supplement regularly may reduce the number of outbreaks and thus the need for topical medications. Of course, you can also use a CBD-infused cream to treat the skin lesions. This may make the second line of defense—oral prescriptions, with their many and varied side effects—less necessary, too.

Natural Partners for CBD

The goal of treating psoriasis is to find the mildest effective treatment to reduce skin turnover and offer relief. CBD certainly fits that bill. Here are a few more things to try:

➤ **GET SOME SUNSHINE.** Exposure to small amounts of sunlight can encourage skin turnover and reduce scaling and inflammation.

➤ **EAT FISH.** The omega-3 fatty acids in fish may also reduce inflammation. Eat more fatty fish, such as salmon or sardines, or take a fish oil supplement.

➤ **RELAX IN A WARM BATH.** Daily baths can help remove dead skin cells and soothe irritated skin, especially if you add nontoxic bath oils, salts, or colloidal oatmeal to the warm (not hot) water. These baths also serve to reduce stress, which can trigger flare-ups. Follow up with a high-quality moisturizer for good measure.

➤ **TAKE NOTES.** Everyone has different triggers, so a great way to discover and avoid yours is to keep a journal about flare-ups. Pay special attention to stress and alcohol consumption, which are common triggers.

SCHIZOPHRENIA

> ➤ Schizophrenia is a serious mental health condition that affects a person's perception of reality.

> ➤ More than 3 million Americans suffer from schizophrenia.

> ➤ Studies show that neuroprotective CBD may reduce the cognitive impairment associated with schizophrenia.

Imagine seeing shadowy creatures lurking in your peripheral vision and hearing them taunt you with cruel words. They tell you to hurt yourself or others, and they crowd out everything else going on around you—school, work, your friends and loved ones. These disturbing hallucinations are as real to someone with schizophrenia as hearing the person next to them speaking. And without proper treatment, it can get worse. CBD may be able to offer those with schizophrenia relief from some of the symptoms so they can live fuller, more independent lives.

Inside Schizophrenia

Schizophrenia is a mental health disorder that causes hallucinations, delusions, and abnormal thinking and behavior. The condition is usually diagnosed when an individual is in the mid to late 20s, but sometimes teenagers are affected. Though scientists do not know what causes schizophrenia, many believe that antipsychotics are the most effective treatment.

CAUSES

Schizophrenia is still a mystery to researchers, but they believe it may be caused by a combination of genetics, brain chemistry, and environment. The neurological differences between those with and without schizophrenia is evident in brain scans. Scientists have been studying the relationship among schizophrenia, the endocannabinoid system, and endocannabinoids for many years.

SYMPTOMS

Symptoms of schizophrenia can vary in severity but usually include:

> **DELUSIONS.** These are beliefs that have no basis in reality, such as believing that you are someone who you are not, or that someone is out to get you.

> **HALLUCINATIONS.** These can affect any of the senses, but typically involve hearing or seeing things that do not exist.

> **DISORGANIZED THINKING.** People with schizophrenia may use meaningless words, or string words together in ways that do not make sense, essentially losing their ability to communicate effectively.

> **DISORGANIZED BEHAVIOR.** This kind of abnormal behavior may include resisting instruction, not responding, moving excessively, or sitting in an unusual position.

> **INABILITY TO FUNCTION.** People with schizophrenia frequently lack personal hygiene, show no emotion, and lose interest in everyday activities.

Top Complications of Schizophrenia

Without proper treatment, schizophrenia can lead to serious and life-altering complications that include:

> Anxiety and obsessive-compulsive disorder

> Depression

> Substance abuse

> Social isolation

> Self-injury

> Inability to attend work or school

> Legal and financial problems

> Homelessness

> Suicide

Who Is at Risk?

Although scientists do not know what causes schizophrenia, they have noticed links between the condition and some factors:

> **FAMILY HISTORY.** Having close family members with schizophrenia can increase risk, as can having an older father.

> **OVERACTIVE IMMUNE SYSTEM.** Chronic inflammation and autoimmune diseases appear to be connected to schizophrenia risk .

> **PREGNANCY AND BIRTH COMPLICATIONS.** Malnutrition and exposure to toxins or viruses *in utero* may play a role.

> **DRUGS.** Taking mind-altering drugs during the teenage years may increase risk.

The CBD Answer

CBD's neuroprotective and immune-balancing properties make it a promising option to include in a schizophrenia treatment plan. It has several of the same effects as common schizophrenia treatments, without harmful side effects.

HOW TO USE IT

Schizophrenia is a serious condition, so consulting with a medical professional about CBD is first and foremost. Keep in mind that THC has been shown to worsen the symptoms of schizophrenia, though some cannabis clinicians believe that nonintoxicating amounts of THC are beneficial.

A Real Problem

Schizophrenia is not just a devastating illness; it can also be a deadly one.

> People with schizophrenia have a higher risk of premature death.

> The number-one cause of premature death in people with schizophrenia is suicide. Another leading cause is overdose.

> Roughly 40 percent of those with schizophrenia go untreated and do not get the help they need.

WHY IT WORKS

Studies have suggested that anandamide, an endocannabinoid produced by the body, may interact with CBD to create an antipsychotic effect. CBD interacts with dopamine receptors in the same communication pathway as do conventional schizophrenia medications. As a neuroprotective compound, CBD may balance neurological functioning by activating receptors in the nervous system. At least one study has shown that it is comparable to an antipsychotic medication but without the often serious side effects.

CBD VERSUS OTHER TREATMENTS

Medications such as antipsychotics are an absolute necessity in treating schizophrenia. Like antipsychotics, CBD interacts with dopamine receptors. CBD also can have similar effects as anti-anxiety and antidepressant meds, which are also used to treat schizophrenia. That means that adding CBD may eventually increase the effectiveness of those medications at lower doses.

Natural Partners for CBD

Schizophrenia is not a condition that can be treated without conventional medicine at this time. However, integrating CBD with other holistic approaches under your prescribing doctor's direction may help:

- ➤ **BE MINDFUL.** Learning to control and quiet the mind by developing a regular meditation practice is an essential tool in combatting mental health issues.

- ➤ **REDUCE INFLAMMATION.** Because schizophrenia has some ties to immune disorders and chronic inflammation, following an anti-inflammatory food plan may help. Replace sugary and

---

The Truth about Schizophrenia Meds

Antipsychotics are serious medications for serious conditions. Unfortunately, these pharmaceuticals come with just as serious side effects, including involuntary jerking movements, muscle spasms, tremors, restlessness, dizziness, and blurred vision. They often cloud consciousness and interfere with clarity of thought.

---

highly processed foods with whole, nutrient-rich foods and be sure to get enough omega-3 fatty acids.

➤ **MOVE YOUR BODY DAILY.** Movement activities can reduce stress and boost feelings of happiness and well-being. That does not necessarily mean hitting the gym or becoming a marathon runner. Activities may include hiking, doing yoga, swimming, and biking.

With a mild, nutty flavor, hemp is easy to enjoy and contains restorative fats, plant-based protein, and numerous vitamins and minerals—all with incredible nutritional and health benefits.

HEMP AS FOOD

Another Powerful Part
of the Cannabis Plant

HOW HEMP MAY FUEL HEALTH

No discussion about the benefits of cannabis would be complete without a look at another beneficial part of the plant—the seeds. Hemp for food comes from the seeds of the plant. Typically consumed raw, these power-packed seeds have incredible nutritional and health benefits.

Hemp Seed Products

A nutritional dynamo, hemp contains restorative fats, plant-based protein, and numerous vitamins and minerals—including magnesium, phosphorus, zinc, potassium, sulfur, and zinc. Hemp is available as various food products:

- Hemp seeds, or hearts
- Hemp oil
- Hemp protein powder
- Hemp flour
- Hemp milk
- Hemp-based snacks

RESTORATIVE FATS

Hemp seeds are vegan-friendly and boast a macronutrient makeup of primarily restorative fats and high-quality protein. Plus, hemp contains three of the essential fatty acids, or EFAs, that the body requires to function optimally—in immune system, heart, and brain health and for many other processes. Because humans do not produce these fats, they must come from food—hence the name *essential* fatty acids. Hemp seeds contain these EFAs:

> ➤ Linoleic acid

> ➤ Alpha-linoleic acid, or ALA

> ➤ Gamma-linoleic acid, or GLA

Hemp seeds features these EFAs in an ideal ratio for health—3:1 omega-6 to omega-3.

PLANT-BASED PROTEIN

Hemp seeds provide a complete protein, meaning it contains all essential amino acids, making it comparable to animal protein sources. Plants rarely contain all amino acids—another positive aspect of the cannabis plant! Protein is, of course, the foundation for all bodily structures and serves as a substrate for hormones and neurotransmitters, as well as the basis for enzymes, which control all biochemical reactions within the body. Another bonus: the digestibility of hemp protein is very good—superior to protein from many grains, nuts, and legumes. The protein that hemp contains is composed of:

> ➤ Edestin (65 percent), which aids in digestion, promotes immune system health, and functions as the backbone of DNA

> ➤ Albumin (35 percent), which helps maintain fluid balance, acts as a transport vessel, and scavenges harmful free radicals

Nutrition Facts for Hemp Seeds

Serving size: 3 tablespoons

Amount Per Serving:

Calories 170

Calories from Fat 120
  Total Fat 14g
  Saturated Fat 1.5g
  Trans Fat 0g
  Polyunsaturated Fat 11g
  Monounsaturated Fat 2g

Cholesterol 0mg

Sodium 0mg

Total Carbohydrate 2g
  Dietary Fiber 1g
  Sugars <1g

Protein 10g

Ingredients: Raw shelled hemp seed

Nourish Your Skin

From lip balm to body wash, beauty companies have found ways to incorporate this ingenious extract into ready-to-use products. One such company has successfully created an entire brand of all-natural bath and beauty products that feature hemp seed oil as the active ingredient. Basically, if you can fit it in your bathroom cabinet, you will find a version of it enriched with hemp seed oil.

How to Eat Hemp

Hemp seeds have a mild, nutty flavor, and just a tablespoon or two can increase your daily nutrient intake. They are easy to add to most meals, so get creative! Here are a few ideas to get you started:

> Top your yogurt bowl with them.

> Mix them into your morning smoothie.

> Sprinkle them on granola or cereal.

> Add them to your soup or salad.

> Blend them into dips and sauces, such as hummus or pesto.

> Use them to make homemade hemp milk for a dairy-free milk alternative.

At a Glance

> CBD oil and hemp seeds come from two different parts of the cannabis plant.

> Hemp seeds have incredible nutritional value, thanks to their fats, protein, vitamins, and minerals.

> Adding just one or two tablespoons to your food each day can improve your health.

> Hemp comes in many food forms (seeds, oil, protein, flour, milk) and can be added to anything from smoothies to salads to dips.

> Finding beauty products with hemp seed oil can boost your overall wellness.

RESOURCES

For more information about cannabis (marijuana and hemp), cannabinoids (including CBD and THC), herbal and botanical medicine, and the endocannabinoid system, check out the following selected resources.

BOOKS

➤ Backes, Michael. *Cannabis Pharmacy: The Practical Guide to Medical Marijuana.* Philadelphia: Running Press, 2017.

➤ Goldstein, Dr. Bonni. *Cannabis Revealed: How the World's Most Misunderstood Plant Is Healing Everything from Chronic Pain to Epilepsy.* Bonni S. Goldstein MD Inc., 2016.

➤ Leinow, Leonard and Juliana Birnbaum. *CBD: A Patient's Guide to Medical Cannabis—Healing Without the High.* Berkeley: North Atlantic Books, 2017.

WEBSITES

➤ **American Botanical Council**
abc.herbalgram.org

➤ **American Herbal Pharmacopoeia**
herbal-ahp.org

➤ **American Herbal Products Association**
ahpa.org

➤ **Hemp Industries Association**
thehia.org

➤ **Holistic Cannabis Academy**
holisticcannabisacademy.com

➤ **International Association for Cannabinoid Medicines**
cannabis-med.org

➤ **International Cannabinoid Research Society**
icrs.co

➤ **National Cannabis Industry Association**
thecannabisindustry.org

> **National Hemp Association**
  nationalhempassociation.org

> **Project CBD**
  projectcbd.com

> **U.S. Hemp Roundtable**
  hempsupporter.com

JOURNAL ARTICLES

> Caramia, G. **"Essential Fatty Acids and Lipid Mediators: Endocannabinoids."** *La Pediatria Medica E Chirurgica* 34, no. 2. (March 2012): 65–72, https://www.ncbi.nlm.nih.gov/pubmed/22730630.

> Di Marzo, V. and F. Piscitelli. **"The Endocannabinoid System and Its Modulation by Phytocannabinoids."** *Neurotherapeutics* 12, no. 4 (October 2015): 692–698, https://www.ncbi.nlm.nih.gov/pubmed/26271952.

> Hampson, A. J., M. Grimaldi, J. Axelrod, and D. Wink. **"Cannabidiol and (-)Delta9-tetrahydrocannabinol Are Neuroprotective Antioxidants."** *Proceedings of the National Academy of Sciences of the United States of America* 95, no. 14 (July 1998): 8268-8273, https://www.ncbi.nlm.nih.gov/pubmed/9653176.

> Iffland, K. and F. Grotenhermen. **"An Update on Safety and Side Effects of Cannabidiol: A Review of Clinical Data and Relevant Animal Studies."** *Cannabis and Cannabinoid Research* 2, no. 1 (June 2017):139–154, https://www.ncbi.nlm.nih.gov/pubmed/28861514.

> Kogan, N. M. and R. Mechoulam. **"Cannabinoids in Health and Disease."** *Dialogues in Clinical Neuroscience* 9, no. 4 (December 2007): 413–430, https://www.ncbi.nlm.nih.gov/pmc/articles/PMC3202504.

> McPartland, J. M., G. W. Guy, and V. Di Marzo. **"Care and Feeding of the Endocannabinoid System: A Systematic Review of Potential Clinical Interventions That Upregulate the Endocannabinoid System,"** *PLoS One.* 9, no. 3 (2014): e89566, https://www.ncbi.nlm.nih.gov/pmc/articles/PMC3951193.

➤ Mouhamed, Y. et al. **"Therapeutic Potential of Medicinal Marijuana: An Educational Primer for Health Care Professionals."** *Drug, Healthcare and Patient Safety* 10 (June 2018): 45–66, https://www.ncbi.nlm.nih.gov/pubmed/29928146.

➤ Naughton, S. S. et al. **"Fatty Acid Modulation of the Endocannabinoid System and the Effect on Food Intake and Metabolism."** *International Journal of Endocrinology* (2013), https://www.hindawi.com/journals/ije/2013/361895.

➤ Russo, E. B. **"Beyond Cannabis: Plants and the Endocannabinoid System."** *Trends in Pharmacological Sciences* 37, no. 7 (July 2016): 594–605, https://www.ncbi.nlm.nih.gov/pubmed/27179600.

➤ Russo, E. B. **"Cannabidiol Claims and Misconceptions."** *Trends in Pharmacological Sciences* 38, no. 3 (March 2017): 198–201, https://www.sciencedirect.com/science/article/pii/S0165614716301869.

➤ Russo, E. B. **"Clinical Endocannabinoid Deficiency (CECD): Can This Concept Explain Therapeutic Benefits of Cannabis in Migraine, Fibromyalgia, Irritable Bowel Syndrome and Other Treatment-Resistant Conditions?"** *Neuroendocrinology Letters* 25, nos. 1–2 (Feb.–Apr. 2004): 31–9, https://www.ncbi.nlm.nih.gov/pubmed/15159679.

➤ Russo, E. B. **"Clinical Endocannabinoid Deficiency Reconsidered: Current Research Supports the Theory in Migraine, Fibromyalgia, Irritable Bowel, and Other Treatment-Resistant Syndromes."** *Cannabis and Cannabinoid Research* 1, no. 1 (July 2016): 154–165, https://www.ncbi.nlm.nih.gov/pubmed/28861491.

➤ Russo, E. B. **"Taming THC: Potential Cannabis Synergy and Phytocannabinoid-Terpenoid Entourage Effects."** *British Journal of Pharmacology* 163, no. 7 (August 2011): 1344–1364, https://www.ncbi.nlm.nih.gov/pmc/articles/PMC3165946.

SCIENTIFIC CONFERENCES

- **Cannabis Science Conference**
  cannabisscienceconference.com

- **CannMed**
  cannmedevents.com

- **Marijuana for Medical Professionals**
  marijuanaformedicalprofessionals.com

- **Patients Out of Time**
  patientsoutoftime.org

For additional resources, visit lauralagano.com

INDEX

holistic approach for, 86

movement activities for, 86

psoriatic, 210, 211

risk factors for, 84–85

symptoms of, 84

ASD. *See Autism spectrum disorder (ASD)*

Ashkenazi Jews, and inflammatory bowel disease, 157

Aspartame

and migraine, 181

and seizures, 142

Asperger's syndrome. *See Autism spectrum disorder (ASD)*

Aspirin, asthma caused by, 88, 89

Asthma, 87–91

adult-onset, 89

allergy-induced, 88

aspirin-induced, 88, 89

causes of, 88–89

cold-induced, 88, 89

deaths from, 87, 90

eczema and, 135, 137

exercise-induced, 88, 89

health care costs of, 87–88

inflammation and, 109, 110

medications for, 90

nocturnal, 89

occupational, 88

prevalence of, 87–88, 109

prevention of, 91

risk factors for, 95

symptoms of, 95

triggers, 88, 91

Atherosclerosis, 151

Atopic dermatitis. *See Eczema*

Attention-deficit hyperactivity disorder (ADHD), 92–97

in adults, 94, 97

associated challenges, 93

CBD for, 95–96

combination, 93

health care costs of, 96

hyperactive-impulsive, 93, 96

inattentive or predominantly inattentive, 93

risk factors for, 93–94

symptoms of, 92–94

Aura, migraine, 182

Autism spectrum disorder (ASD), vi–vii, 26, 98–103

adults with, 99

causes of, 99

CBD for, 99, 101–102

complications of, 101

definition of, 98

and epilepsy, 100, 102, 139, 140

inflammation and, 109

medications for, 99

prevalence of, 98

risk factors for, 100–101

symptoms of, 99, 100

Autoimmune disease. *See also Inflammatory bowel disease (IBD); Multiple sclerosis (MS); Psoriasis*

and bone loss, 195

inflammation and, 108, 135

and schizophrenia risk, 217

Avoidance, in PTSD, 201

B

Bacterial overgrowth, and irritable bowel syndrome, 168

Balance. *See Homeostasis*

Balms, 35

Barometric pressure, and migraine, 181

Bath products

CBD-infused, 31

hemp seed oil in, 224

Baths, for psoriasis, 214

Beauty products
CBD-infused, 30–32, 43
hemp seed oil in, 224
Behavior
in autism, 100
disorganized, in schizophrenia, 216
Benzodiazepines, 77
Benzoyl peroxide, 60
Berberine, 133
Beta-caryophyllene, 19
Beta-myrcene, 19
BHA, 35
BHT, 35
Bioavailability, 33–34, 37, 46
definition of, 36
factors affecting, 36
Biofeedback
for chronic pain, 117
for irritable bowel syndrome, 172
Biotin, for multiple sclerosis
management, 189
Biphasic effects, of CBD, 40
Bipolar disorder, 125
Bisphosphonates, 195
Blackheads, 57
Bladder function, multiple
sclerosis and, 185
Blindness
diabetes and, 130
glaucoma and, 148, 149
Bliss molecule. *See Anandamide*
Bloating, premenstrual
syndrome and, 206
Blood glucose. *See Blood sugar*
Blood pressure
CBD and, 154
high. *See Hypertension*
Blood sugar, 129, 131
and epilepsy management, 142

factors affecting, 133
management of, 82
and seizures, 139
tracking, 132
Blue Dream, 15
Body aches, inflammation and, 110
Body products, CBD-infused, 31
Bone density loss, 26, 176.
See also Osteoporosis
triggers, 195
Bone health, 194, 197–198
Bone strength, 26
Bosellia, 146
Bowel function, multiple
sclerosis and, 185
Brain, inflammation of,
and epilepsy, 139
Brain chemistry
and depression, 124
and premenstrual syndrome, 206
Brain fog
fibromyalgia and, 144
premenstrual syndrome and, 206
Brain health, promotion of, 72, 77–78
Brain injury, and epilepsy, 140–141
Brain tumor, and epilepsy, 139
Breathing exercises
and ADHD management, 97
anti-inflammatory effects of, 112
for nausea, 193
Bronchodilator, CBD as, and
asthma treatment, 89, 90
Brown fat, 129
Butterbur, for migraine treatment, 183

C

Caffeine, 67
abstinence from, and PTSD
management, 204
and insomnia, 162–163

Hydration, and skin conditions, 31

Hydrocortisone, 136

Hygiene, and heart disease, 153

Hypertension, 26
  corticosteroids and, 111
  diabetes and, 130
  and glaucoma, 149
  and heart disease, 153
  sleep deprivation and, 162

Hyperthyroidism, and bone loss, 195

Hysterectomy, 174

I

IBD. *See Inflammatory bowel disease (IBD)*

IBS. *See Irritable bowel syndrome (IBS)*

Ibuprofen, 111
  asthma caused by, 88
  for chronic pain, 116
  and inflammatory bowel
    disease, 157–158

Illness
  and chronic pain, 115
  and depression, 123

Immune system, 30
  CBD and, 27
  and schizophrenia, 217

Inactivity
  and diabetes, 130
  and fibromyalgia, 145
  and heart disease, 153
  and osteoporosis, 196

Individualized medicine, 39–40

Infection(s)
  and Alzheimer's disease, 70
  and appetite loss, 80
  corticosteroids and, 111
  and epilepsy, 139, 141
  of heart, 152
  and heart disease, 153

and irritable bowel syndrome, 168

and multiple sclerosis, 186

and psoriasis, 212

skin, 119

Inflammation. *See also*
Chronic inflammation
  acute, 108
  and appetite loss, 81
  CBD for, 25
  and depression, 123
  and insomnia, 163–165
  of skin, 118
  and skin conditions, 27, 30
  sugar and, 45

Inflammatory bowel disease
  (IBD), 156–160
  and bone loss, 195
  causes of, 157
  CBD for, 158–159
  in children, 159
  costs of, 158
  holistic approach for, 159–160
  vs. irritable bowel syndrome, 156
  and multiple sclerosis, 186
  in pets, CBD for, 50
  prevalence of, 156
  risk factors for, 157–158
  symptoms of, 157

Ingredients
  artificial
    and autism, 102–103
    and hyperactivity, 95, 97
    to avoid, 35, 45
    in pet products, 51

Injury. *See also Head injury/trauma*
  and arthritis, 85
  and chronic pain, 114
  and fibromyalgia, 145

Insomnia, 161–172, 176

and Alzheimer's disease, 71

and epilepsy treatment, 141

and fibromyalgia, 146

and multiple sclerosis, 188

for pets, 51

and schizophrenia, 217, 218

Neurotransmitters

CBD and, 18

and depression, 124

Niacin, and heart health, 155

Nickel allergy, 121

Nightmares, in PTSD, 200

Night sweats, menopause and, 175

Nocturia, 166

Nodules, 57

Nonsteroidal antiinflammatory drugs (NSAIDs), 111

for chronic pain, 116

and inflammatory bowel disease, 157–158

Nuclear receptors, CBD and, 21

Numbness, multiple sclerosis and, 185

Nutrient deficiency, and depression, 123

Nutrition. *See also Food(s)*

in autism treatment, 102–103

and brain health, 77

and lung health, 91

and osteoporosis, 196

Nutritional supplements, 28. *See also Supplements*

O

Obesity. *See also Overweight*

and arthritis, 85

health effects of, 111

and heart disease, 26, 153

and inflammation, 109, 111

and menopausal complications, 175

and premenstrual syndrome, 207

prevalence of, 111

and psoriasis, 213

Obsessive-compulsive disorder (OCD), 74, 77

Occupation

and contact dermatitis, 119

and PTSD risk, 201

Occupational asthma, 88

Oils. *See also Essential oils*

CBD, topical, 35

Ointments, CBD, 35

Omega-3 fatty acids, 60–61

and ADHD management, 97

and bone health, 197

and eye health, 150

and heart health, 155

and multiple sclerosis management, 188

for psoriasis, 214

in schizophrenia management, 219

Opioid addiction, 62, 117

Opioid epidemic, 116, 117

Opioids

abstinence from, and PTSD management, 204

for chronic pain, 116

Oral products, CBD, 33–34, 43

for arthritis, 85

for eczema, 136

Organic products, 44–45

for pets, 51

Orgasm

anti-inflammatory effects of, 112

and anxiety management, 78

Orphan receptors, CBD and, 20

O'Shaughnessy, William Brooke, 8

Osteoarthritis, 83–84. *See also Arthritis*

Osteoporosis, 3, 26, 176, 194–198

ACKNOWLEDGMENTS

My career in nutrition, cannabis, and all things holistic happened because of the people around me, the relationships in my life. At the end of the day, what's more important than your peeps, your tribe?

The groundwork for this book was laid by a few key people in the cannabis world. Raphael Mechoulam—whom I was lucky enough to interview for *Holistic Primary Care*—sparked curiosity about the cannabis plant when he isolated THC, did the initial studies about CBD and seizures, and later revealed the endocannabinoid system. Vincenzo Di Manzo, John McPartland, and Ethan Russo asked the questions and posed the theories, inciting us to perk up and rediscover a plant. Thank you to the pioneers.

Mary Lynn Mathre was the first healthcare practitioner I met who knew about cannabis. She more than knew: Mary Lynn is the de facto inventor of cannabis education, as the founder of Patients Out of Time, a clinical cannabis conference. That is where I met Debbie Malka, who has been teaching patients about cannabis for over two decades. Both women are extraordinary healers. They, as well as Ethan Russo, have generously given their time and expertise to the writing of this book.

As the cofounder (along with Donna Shields) and education director of an online cannabis education program, I have had the opportunity to meet a number of incredible teachers who helped review material in this book: Joe Cohen, Oleg MaryAcres, Lex Pelger, Michele Ross, and John Roulac. These are all incredible minds who have not been satisfied with the status quo—thankfully. Without them, the work of ridding the world of cannaphobia could not happen.

My integrative nutrition colleagues have always spurred me on, encouraging me to explore and learn. Kathie Swift, Geri Brewster, and Vicki Kobliner are three of the most intelligent and caring individuals I have ever known. These are the professionals who have literally changed the way nutrition is practiced and opened our eyes to the impacts of food on autism, Alzheimer's, ADHD, and many other conditions. Without them, we would still be talking about the Food Guide Pyramid.

In my learning journey with Isabella, I studied functional medicine with the phenomenal Jeff Bland, Patrick Hanaway (who explained Isabella's genetic results to me), and so many others who were not satisfied with what was. Perhaps top among them is Hyla Cass, a true pioneer who offered her encouragement and expertise in the writing of this book. Tanya Adams provided constant counsel throughout the research and writing process. I could not have done this without her. Much gratitude to Hyla and Tanya.

Then there is Bruce Lubin, who recognized the importance of communicating the benefits of CBD, and my editor Jennifer Leight, who may be the most patient person on the planet. Enormous gratitude goes out to Margaret Woodwell, an incredible researcher and communicator of all things health and wellness. Thank you for believing in cannabis and helping to rid the world of cannaphobia.

Writing a book is a stress-filled experience (that is when CBD comes in handy!). Throughout the process, I relied on the guidance and support of a few old friends. You know who you are. Names are not needed. All my love and devotion to my family—Victoria, Isabella, Zachary, and Stephen, who kept the ship afloat.

ABOUT THE AUTHOR

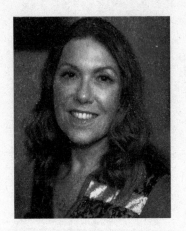 **LAURA LAGANO, MS, RDN, CDN,** is a nutrition, health, and cannabis educator, cofounder and education director of the Holistic Cannabis Academy, and contributing writer for *Holistic Primary Care* and *Kitchen Toke*. She holds a bachelor of science degree in dietetics from SUNY Oneonta and a master's degree in nutrition education from Columbia University, where she is currently a doctoral candidate. As an integrative clinical nutritionist, Laura has a private practice and consulting business based in Hoboken, New Jersey, where she lives with her husband and three kids. Laura can be reached at lauralagano.com.

NOTES

NOTES

NOTES

NOTES